T0328828

Curbside Consultation
in Knee Arthroplasty

49 Clinical Questions

CURBSIDE CONSULTATION IN ORTHOPEDICS
SERIES

SERIES EDITOR, BERNARD R. BACH, JR., MD

Curbside Consultation
in Knee Arthroplasty

49 Clinical Questions

EDITED BY

Craig J. Della Valle, MD
Assistant Professor of Orthopaedic Surgery
Rush University Medical Center
Chicago, Illinois

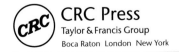

CRC Press
Taylor & Francis Group
Boca Raton London New York

CRC Press is an imprint of the
Taylor & Francis Group, an **informa** business

First published 2008 by SLACK Incorporated

Published 2024 by CRC Press
2385 NW Executive Center Drive, Suite 320, Boca Raton FL 33431

and by CRC Press
4 Park Square, Milton Park, Abingdon, Oxon, OX14 4RN

CRC Press is an imprint of Taylor & Francis Group, LLC

© 2008 Taylor & Francis Group, LLC

Library of Congress Cataloging-in-Publication Data

Curbside consultation in knee arthroplasty : 49 clinical questions / edited by Craig J. Della Valle.
    p. ; cm.
  Includes bibliographical references and index.
  ISBN 978-1-55642-824-1 (softcover : alk. paper) 1. Knee--Surgery--Miscellanea. 2. Total knee replace-ment--Miscellanea. I. Della Valle, Craig J.
  [DNLM: 1. Knee Joint--surgery. 2. Arthroplasty--methods. WE 870 C975 2008]

RD561.C82 2008
617.5′82059--dc22

                    2007047476

ISBN: 9781556428241 (pbk)
ISBN: 9781003523581 (ebk)

DOI: 10.1201/9781003523581

Dedication

To my parents, Joan and John, for their unwavering support.

Contents

SECTION I: PREOPERATIVE QUESTIONS

SECTION II: INTRAOPERATIVE QUESTIONS

SECTION III: POSTOPERATIVE QUESTIONS

SECTION IV: REVISION QUESTIONS

Acknowledgments

Many thanks to Ashley Racemacher for her assistance.

—*CJD*

About the Editor

Craig J. Della Valle, MD is an Adult Reconstructive Surgeon who focuses on Total Hip and Knee Arthroplasty at Rush University Medical Center in Chicago, IL. He specializes in complex primary and revision surgery as well as unicompartmental arthroplasty of the knee and hip resurfacing. Dr. Della Valle completed his residency at the Hospital for Joint Diseases in New York City and his fellowship in adult reconstructive surgery at Rush. In addition to his clinical duties, he is involved in numerous clinical research projects. Dr. Della Valle serves as an Associate Professor of Orthopaedic Surgery at Rush University Medical Center.

Contributing Authors

Michael Archibeck, MD
New Mexico Center for Joint Replacement
  Surgery
New Mexico Orthopaedics
Albuquerque, NM

Regina Barden, RN, BSN
Rush University Medical Center
Chicago, IL

Robert L. Barrack, MD
Washington University School of Medicine
Barnes-Jewish Hospital
St. Louis, MO

Keith R. Berend, MD
New Albany Surgical Hospital
Ohio State University
New Albany, OH

Richard A. Berger, MD
Rush University Medical Center
Chicago, IL

Daniel J. Berry, MD
Mayo Clinic
Rochester, MN

Hari P. Bezwada, MD
University of Pennsylvania School of
  Medicine
PENN Orthopaedics
Pennsylvania Hospital
Philadelphia, PA

Robert E. Booth, Jr., MD
Pennsylvania Hospital
University of Pennsylvania School of
  Medicine
Philadelphia, PA

Kevin J. Bozic, MD, MBA
UCSF Department of Orthopaedic Surgery
  Institute for Health Policy Studies
San Francisco, CA

Thomas E. Brown, MD,
University of Virginia
Charlottesville, VA

R. Stephen J. Burnett, BSc, MD, FRCS(C),
  Dipl. ABOS
Royal Jubilee Victoria Hospital
Victoria, BC

Cory L. Calendine, MD
The Bone & Joint Clinic
Franklin, TN

Mark D. Campbell, MD
The Core Institute
Anthem, AZ

Diego Cardona, MD
Orthopedic Institute at Mercy Hospital
Miami, FL

Seann Carr, MD
University of Chicago Medical Center
Chicago, IL

Kim Chandler, RN
Rush University Medical Center
Chicago, IL

John C. Clohisy, MD
Washington University
St. Louis, MO

Quan Jun Cui, MD, MS
University of Virginia
Charlottesville, VA

Fred Cushner, MD
Insall Scott Kelly® Institute
New York, NY

Carl Deirmengian, MD
3B Orthopaedics
Philadelphia, PA

Paul E. Di Cesare, MD
UC Davis Medical Center
Sacramento, CA

Frank R. DiMaio, MD
Winthrop—University Hospital
Mineola, NY
State University of New York, Health
  Science Center at Stony Brook
Stony Brook, NY

Mark Dumonski, MD
Rush University Medical Center
Chicago, IL

Andrew A. Freiberg, MD
Massachusetts General Hospital
Harvard Medical School
Yawkey Center For Outpatient Care
Boston, MA

Kevin B. Fricka, MD
The Anderson Orthopaedic Clinic
Alexandria, VA

Donald Garbuz, MD, FRCSC
University of British Columbia
Vancouver, BC

Allan E. Gross, MD, FRCSC, O.Ont.
University of Toronto
Mount Sinai Hospital
Toronto, Ontario

Mark A. Hartzband, MD
Hackensack University Medical Center,
Hackensack, NJ
Hartzband Joint Replacement Institute
Paramus, NJ

Raphael C. Y. Hau, MBBS, FRACS
University of British Columbia
Vancouver, BC

Richard Illgen II, MD
University of Wisconsin Hospital and
   Clinics
Madison, WI

Feridon Jaberi, MD
Rothman Institute at Thomas Jefferson
   University
Philadelphia, PA

Joshua J. Jacobs, MD
Rush University Medical Center
Chicago, IL

David J. Jacofsky, MD
The Center for Orthopedic Research and
   Education
Phoenix, AZ

Harpal Singh Khanuja, MD
Johns Hopkins University
Baltimore, MD

Gregg R. Klein, MD
Hackensack University Medical Center
Hackensack, NJ
Hartzband Joint Replacement Institute
Paramus, NJ

Richard S. Laskin, MD
Hospital for Special Surgery
Weil Medical College of Cornell University
New York, NY

Carlos Lavernia, MD
Orthopedic Institute at Mercy Hospital
Miami, FL

Seth S. Leopold, MD
University of Washington
Seattle, Washington

Brett Levine, MD, MS
Midwest Orthopaedic Center
Peoria, IL

Jay R. Lieberman, MD
New England Musculoskeletal Institute
University of Connecticut Health Center
Farmington, CT

Jess H. Lonner, MD
Booth Bartolozzi Balderston Orthopaedics
Pennsylvania Hospital
Philadelphia Center for Minimally
   Invasive Knee Surgery
Philadelphia, PA

Steven Lyons, MD
Florida Orthopaedic Institute
Tampa, FL

William Macaulay, MD
College of Physicians & Surgeons
Center for Hip and Knee Replacement
   (CHKR)
New York Presbyterian Hospital at
   Columbia University
New York, NY

David Manning, MD
University of Chicago Medical Center
Chicago, IL

Amanda Marshall, MD
University of Texas Health Science Center
   at San Antonio
San Antonio, TX

Bassam A. Masri, MD, FRCSC
University of British Columbia
Vancouver, BC

R. Michael Meneghini, MD
Joint Replacement Surgeons of Indiana
    Research Foundation
St. Vincent Center for Joint Replacement
Indianapolis, IN

William Mihalko, MD, PhD
University of Virginia
Charlottesville, VA

Patrick M. Morgan, MD
University of Minnesota
Minneapolis, MN

Mohammad Namazian, DO
Kaiser Permanente Medical Center
Fontana, CA

David G. Nazarian, MD
Booth Bartolozzi Balderston Orthopaedics
Pennsylvania Hospital
Philadelphia, PA

Javad Parvizi MD, FRCS
Rothman Institute at Thomas Jefferson
    University
Philadelphia, PA

Jeffery L. Pierson, MD
Joint Replacement Surgeons of Indiana
    Research Foundation
St. Vincent Center for Joint Replacement
Indianapolis, IN

Wayne G. Paprosky, MD
Rush University Medical Center
Chicago, IL

Michael D. Reis, MD
University of California, San Francisco
San Francisco, CA

Aaron G. Rosenberg, MD
Rush University Medical Center
Chicago, IL

Scott D. Ruhlman, MD
University of Washington
Seattle, WA

Oleg Safir, MD, FRCSC
University of Toronto
Mount Sinai Hospital
Toronto, Ontario

Khaled Saleh, MD, MSc, FRCSC
University of Virginia
Charlottesville, VA

Shanon M. Sara
University of Washington
Seattle, WA

Mark F. Schinsky, MD
Castle Orthopaedics & Sports Medicine, SC
Aurora, IL

Giles R. Scuderi, MD
Insall Scott Kelly Institute
Albert Einstein College of Medicine
New York, NY

Alexander Siegmeth, FRCS(Tr&Orth)
Vancouver General Hospital
Vancouver, BC

Scott M. Sporer, MD, MS
Rush University Medical Center
Chicago, IL
Central Dupage Hospital
Winfield, IL

Matthew Squire, MD, MS
University of Wisconsin Hospital and
    Clinics
Madison, WI

Steven Stuchin, MD
NYU Hospital for Joint Diseases
New York, NY

Kelly G. Vince, MD, FRCS
Keck School of Medicine of the University
    of Southern California
Los Angeles, CA

Walter Virkus, MD
Rush University Medical Center
Chicago, IL

Steven H. Weeden, MD
Texas Hip and Knee Center
Fort Worth, TX

Markus A. Wimmer, PhD
Rush University Medical Center
Chicago, IL

Foreword

Personal experience is a priceless asset in the hands of the talented surgeon. This book harnesses that knowledge and uses it as a learning tool for the practicing orthopedic surgeon. Structured in the form of questions on subjects that a practitioner is bound to encounter in the course of his daily routine, the book strives to provide realistic and straightforward answers. There are 49 such questions—each put together in the form of a chapter written in an informal style—with only a minimal and essential list of references and a great deal of personal know-how.

As an experienced educator and total knee replacement surgeon, I found the questions relevant and very well selected. They cover the field in almost a comprehensive manner including preoperative decisions and indications, pearls of surgical technique, difficult problems in revision surgery, the management of postoperative complications, and many other subjects the surgeon is bound to encounter in the course of his practice. The approach to writing gives the reader the feeling of direct communication with the expert, of a real "curbside consult," and thus provides the opportunity for a superior learning experience.

Dr. Della Valle and his collaborators have done an excellent job in making available a practical tool of widespread relevance. It certainly belongs in every total knee replacement surgeon's library where it will provide an easily available source of practical knowledge.

— *Jorge Galante, MD*
Chicago, Illinois

SECTION I

PREOPERATIVE QUESTIONS

How Do You Decide When a Patient Is "Ready" for a Total Knee Replacement? Is There a Downside to Waiting Until They Have More Severe Disease?

Carlos Lavernia, MD
Diego Cardona, MD

The exact time in the disease process at which point total knee arthroplasty (TKA) should be performed is unclear and the indications for surgery vary considerably between surgeons. The standard philosophy taught at orthopedic residencies has traditionally emphasized surgical intervention only when the patient has rest and night pain; patients were instructed to seek surgery only if there disability was extreme. This premise has been questioned and reformulated based on a series of scientific papers demonstrating the disadvantages of waiting until disease progression is severe. To date, however, no proven evidence-based indicators exist as to precisely when is the optimal time for surgical intervention.[1] While we as surgeons face complex decisions as to when it is appropriate to recommend surgery, many patients cite fear of major surgery as reason for delaying operative intervention.[2]

Our initial approach in treating patients with knee arthritis is to offer them nonoperative alternatives including the use of acetaminophen, anti-inflammatory medications, physical therapy, and intra-articular injections (corticosteroids and hyaluronic acid). Once these interventions have failed and pain that interferes with the patient's activities of daily living is experienced, a mutual decision is made between the surgeon and the patient to proceed with surgery based on an analysis of the risks and benefits of surgical intervention. Patients expectations of TKA should be discussed extensively at this

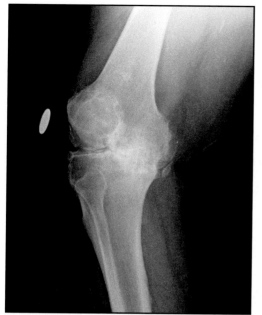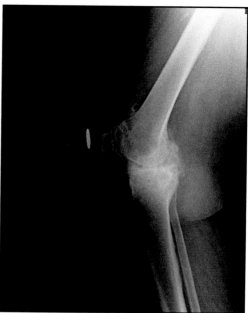

Figure 1-1. AP and lateral radiographs of a 67-year-old patient with moderate right knee pain despite severe radiographic changes; the patient refused surgical treatment.

point, as they have been shown to heavily influence the final outcome.[3] In rare cases radiographic evidence of severe bone loss, substantial angular deformity, flexion contracture, or stiffness can be good indications for TKA in the absence of severe radiographic changes. It is critical to remember, however, that radiographic evidence of arthritis alone is not a good indication for surgery and likewise some patients can present with only mild radiographic changes but severe pain and after failure of nonoperative treatment are appropriate indications for TKA (Figures 1-1 and 1-2).

Attempts are being made to quantitate the process of deciding when surgery is indicated. We have analyzed a cohort of patients and divided them into two groups according to the degree of functional disability at the time of the surgery. Group 1 included patients with preoperative WOMAC scores greater than 51 (severe/extreme compromise); group 2 included patients with scores of 51 or less (mild or moderate compromise). Both of these instruments measure quality of life in patients. Scores for the SF-36 and QWB (Quality of Well Being Index) were prospectively followed for three years, at the end of which a clear distinction was observed.

Those patients who initially exhibited a greater compromise scored worse than the group that initially exhibited less compromise.[4] Similarly, Garbuz et al observed that the odds of achieving a better than expected postoperative functional outcome decreased by 8% for each month that patients waited for surgery.[5] In addition to the risk of a compromised outcome, there is an economic cost to waiting as well. Fielden et al demonstrated that the average cost of waiting 5 months exceeds $2500.00 per person in miscellaneous costs.[6] Based on this data, we do not feel that patients should wait until their symptoms or clinical disability become intolerable in order to proceed with surgery. As with most clinical entities, the odds of achieving complete success improve if the disease is treated

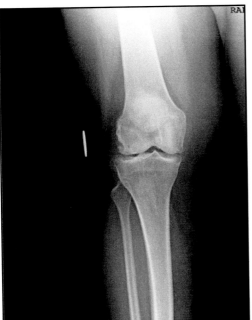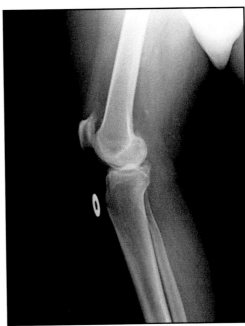

Figure 1-2. 73-year-old patient with severe right knee pain recalcitrant to nonoperative treatment with mild radiographic changes who was scheduled for a TKA.

before irreparable damage has been done. The musculoskeletal system is no exception, and damage caused to muscles, tendons, and ligaments surrounding an arthritic knee should not be allowed to cross the threshold of reparability obtained with surgery.

References

1. Gaudet M-C, Feldman DE, Rossignol M, et al. The wait for total hip replacement in patients with osteoarthritis. *Can J Surg.* 2007; 50(2):101-109.
2. Clark JP, Hudak PL, Hawker GA, Coyte PC, Mahomed NN, Kreder HJ, Wright JG. The moving target: a qualitative study of elderly patients' decision-making regarding total joint replacement surgery. *J Bone Joint Surg Am.* 2004;86-A(7):1366-1374.
3. Mahomed NN, Liang MH, Cook EF, Daltroy LH, Fortin PR, Fossel AH, Katz JN. The importance of patient expectations in predicting functional outcomes after total joint arthroplasty. *J Rheumatol.* 2002;29(6): 1273-1279.
4. Lavernia C, Hernandez VH, D'Apuzzo M, Rossi M, Lee DP. Primary arthroplasty: should we wait as much as possible? In: *American Academy of Orthopedic Surgery Meeting*, paper 001. Chicago, Illinois, 2006.
5. Garbuz DS, Xu M, Duncan CP, Masri BA, Sobolev B. Delays worsen quality of life outcome of primary total hip arthroplasty. *Clin Orthop Relat Res.* 2006;447:79-84.
6. Fielden JM, Cumming JM, Horne JG, Devane PA, Slack A, Gallagher LM. Waiting for hip arthroplasty: economic costs and health outcomes. *J Arthroplasty.* 2005;20(8):990-997.

I Have a Patient That Looks Like They May Be a Candidate for Either a Unicompartmental Knee Replacement, a Total Knee Replacement, or an HTO. How Do I Decide Among These Options?

Michael Archibeck, MD

The younger the patient with osteoarthritis of the knee, the greater the potential benefits in postponing the need for surgical intervention. Thus, nonsurgical management should be the initial approach in these patients. Assuming nonsurgical management has been inadequate, several surgical options can be considered. These include high tibial osteotomy, unicompartmental knee replacement, and total knee replacement. I will discuss my evaluation of these patients and the indications for each surgical option below.

The initial evaluation includes a thorough history including a discussion of the location, character, and factors that exacerbate the symptoms. I ask about patellofemoral symptoms and their severity (pain with stairs, prolonged sitting with the knee flexed, squatting, hills, etc). I will ask about prior nonsurgical or surgical treatment the patient has undergone. Physical examination includes an assessment of gait (antalgic component, alignment, and any varus thrust); sitting exam includes palpation of the patellofemoral joint with flexion and extension; finally the supine portion of the exam includes an evaluation of the hip, palpation of the joint line, ligamentious stability, range of motion, and any special tests. Neurovascular assessment should be performed as well. Radiographic evaluation includes a weight bearing AP view, a flexion PA weight bearing view, a full-length weight bearing image of the extremity, a lateral, and a merchant view. Occasionally additional imaging may be needed if significant instability is present or mechanical symptoms are suggestive of meniscal pathology.

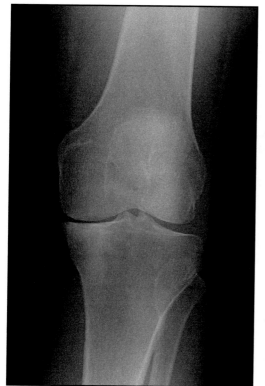

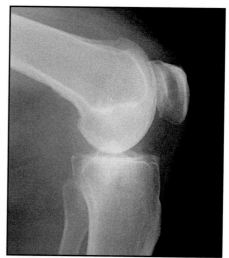

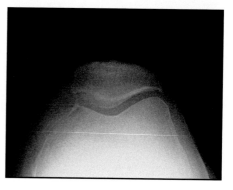

Figure 2-1. These radiographs demonstrate the appearance of osteoarthritis primarily of the medial compartment with associated mechanical varus alignment.

The use of high tibial osteotomy (closing or opening wedge) has diminished during the last decade despite a well-documented record of success over a 7 to 10 year period in appropriately selected patients.[1] The decreased use of this procedure largely comes from higher complication rates compared to alternatives, increased popularity of unicompartmental knee arthroplasty (UKA), increased willingness of surgeons to offer total knee arthroplasty (TKA) to younger patients, and the technical demands of the procedure. I believe there remains a patient population that is best served by high tibial osteotomy. However, the patient needs to be well educated as to the potential complications and the expectations regarding incomplete pain relief and the likely need for subsequent TKA in the future. In order for me to consider a high tibial osteotomy (HTO) the patient's pain needs to be well localized to the medial aspect of the knee and correlate well with radiographic findings (Figure 2-1). My indications for such an osteotomy include the following:

1. Less than 40 years old.

2. Very active work or lifestyle.

3. Typically male.

4. Typically large patient.

5. Varus malalignment with medial compartment disease.

6. Noninflammatory arthritis.

7. Well maintained range of motion (90 or more degree arc of motion).

8. In conjunction with cartilage restoration efforts (cartilage transplantation, meniscal transplantation) association with varus malalignment.

Unicompartmental knee arthroplasty (UKA) has increased in its popularity with improved reported clinical results,[2] less invasive techniques,[3] and patient satisfaction with the procedure. In comparison to high tibial osteotomy it has been shown to have fewer complications and a higher initial success rate. In comparison to TKA, UKA has been shown to have a superior patient preference, fewer complications, to be less invasive, and restore more normal kinematics of the knee. However, the literature remains sparse with respect to its use in young active patients and should be used with caution in this population. My indications for UKA include the following:

1. Isolated medial or lateral noninflammatory disease.

2. Typically over 65 years of age.

3. Less than 80 to 90 kg.

4. Limited deformity (less than 5 degrees of varus or 10 degrees of valgus).

5. No or minimal patellofemoral disease or symptoms.

6. The absence of significant tibiofemoral subluxation.

7. An intact ACL.

While some surgeons have pushed the limits of UKA in younger, heavier, more active patients, the data has been inferior to that published in the more idealized patient and should be performed with caution and an understanding of the goals of the procedure as a temporizing measure.[4]

TKA has demonstrated good survivorship and functional results in a variety of studies in young patients.[5,6] The benefits of TKA in these patients include its more complete pain relief in patients with bi- or tricompartmental knee arthritis, its ability to correct significant deformity, and high level of surgeon comfort and familiarity. Concerns regarding its use in young active patients include issues of limited longevity, polyethylene wear and osteolysis, and more complex salvage than HTO or UKA. My indications for TKA in young, active patients include:

1. Advanced bi- or tricompartmental disease.

2. Inflammatory disease.

3. Significant deformity.

4. Tibiofemoral subluxation.

5. Diffuse pain, despite localized radiographic changes.

While the decision-making process can by quite difficult for patient and surgeon alike, a thorough understanding of the contraindications for each procedure often simplify the task. In my experience, most patients suffer from tricompartmental disease and surgical treatment is limited to TKA. In the occasional patient with unicompartmental disease and localized symptoms, HTO or UKA can be considered. The choice, in my mind, is then based on the amount of deformity, the size and activity level of the patient, and patient preference.

References

1. Billings A, Scott DF, Camargo MP, Hofmann AA. High tibial osteotomy with a calibrated osteotomy guide, rigid internal fixation, and early motion. Long-term follow-up. *J Bone Joint Surg Am.* 2000;82(1):70-79.
2. Berger RA, Meneghini RM, Jacobs JJ, Sheinkop MB, Della Valle CJ, Rosenberg AG, Galante JO. Results of unicompartmental knee arthroplasty at a minimum of ten years of follow-up. *J Bone Joint Surg Am.* 2005;87(5):999-1006.
3. Pandit H, Jenkins C, Barker K, Dodd CA, Murray DW. The Oxford medial unicompartmental knee replacement using a minimally-invasive approach. *J Bone Joint Surg Br.* 2006;88(1):54-60.
4. Pennington DW, Swienckowski JJ, Lutes WB, Drake GN. Unicompartmental knee arthroplasty in patients sixty years of age or younger. *J Bone Joint Surg Am.* 2003; 85-A(10):1968-1973.
5. Gill GS, Chan KC, Mills DM. 5- to 18-year follow-up study of cemented total knee arthroplasty for patients 55 years old or younger. *J Arthroplasty.* 1997;12(1):49-54.
6. Lonner JH, Hershman S, Mont M, Lotke PA. Total knee arthroplasty in patients 40 years of age and younger with osteoarthritis. *Clin Orthop Relat Res.* 2000;380:85-90.

I Have a Patient With a Deformity of the Distal Femur and Arthritis of the Knee. Should I Do an Osteotomy to Correct the Deformity at the Time of Total Knee Arthroplasty?

Jess H. Lonner, MD

Component fixation, component and limb alignment, and soft tissue balancing contribute to success after total knee arthroplasty. My preference is to implant the femoral and tibial components perpendicular to the mechanical axis of the femur and tibia, respectively. In the setting of femoral deformity from metabolic diseases such as Rickets, Paget's disease, fracture malunion, or previous distal femoral osteotomy, a decision needs to be made about whether a total knee arthroplasty can be performed in a traditional fashion, albeit perhaps with the use of extramedullary instrumentation, or whether a staged or simultaneous femoral osteotomy is necessary, to ensure that the femoral component is implanted with appropriate alignment and without compromising collateral ligament balance. Complex imbalance of the collateral ligaments can result in the presence of large extra-articular deformities, when trying to balance the ligaments entirely within the joint with soft tissue releases. Femoral malunions that are proximal to the isthmus will rarely compromise collateral ligament origins when resecting the distal femur perpendicular to the mechanical axis because these deformities are often compensated well by the hip. However, with more distal deformities, standard resection of the distal femur may result in cutting the collateral ligament attachment. In such cases, a corrective osteotomy is prudent (Figures 3-1 and 3-2). Simultaneous corrective osteotomy and total knee arthroplasty is safe and effective with predictably good results.[1-4]

Figure 3-1. Fifteen degree supracondylar fracture malunion and degenerative knee arthritis. Planned resection of the distal femur perpendicular to the mechanical axis would compromise the origin of the lateral collateral ligament.

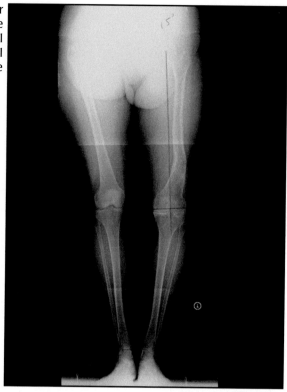

There are trigonometric formulas which can be used to calculate whether the deformities need to be corrected prior to total knee arthroplasty,[4] but I use a more rudimentary method. A full-length weight bearing radiograph of the entire lower extremity, from the hip to the ankle, is obtained. Draw the mechanical axis of the femur from the center of the femoral head to the center of the knee. Then draw a perpendicular line at the planned level of resection of the distal femur. If the templated resection compromises the epicondylar attachment of the lateral or medial collateral ligaments, then a corrective osteotomy is necessary. If the deformity is small, or far from the knee, then the resection is less likely to compromise the collateral ligament attachment. In smaller deformities, after resecting the distal femur and implanting the trial components, the soft tissues can be released in a traditional fashion to balance the medial and lateral sleeves. In general, a coronal deformity of at least 15 degrees or a sagittal deformity of 20 degrees or more (particularly when distal to the isthmus), needs to be corrected by osteotomy.

The technique of corrective osteotomy, the method of fixation, and whether the osteotomy is staged with or performed simultaneous with total knee arthroplasty depend collectively on factors such as the size and location of the deformity, medical status of the patient, and surgeon preference. Locked femoral nailing or compression plate fixation are effective fixation methods. Fixation with a press fit stem extension from the femoral component of the total knee arthroplasty is another effective means, although compression of the osteotomy may be slightly more difficult by this method. Two osteotomy options include a closing wedge in the plane of the deformity or an oblique osteotomy, orthogonal to the malunion so that the bone can be rotated on itself and then rigidly fixed.

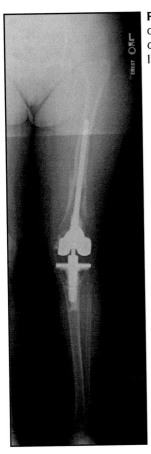

Figure 3-2. Successful oblique corrective osteotomy and simultaneous total knee arthroplasty have been performed, with correction of the mechanical axis of the femur and maintenance of collateral ligament stability.

A radiolucent table and a sterile tourniquet are used. Corrective osteotomies are performed with the assistance of fluoroscopic imaging to assess the location and extent of correction. If a plate or retrograde nail are used to fix the osteotomy, access to the intramedullary canal is eliminated and, therefore, extramedullary techniques need to be used, with or without computer navigation to resect the distal femur. If a press fit stem extension on the femoral component is used to secure the osteotomy, then after the osteotomy is performed, provisional manual fixation of the osteotomy is held followed by reaming of the canals both distal and proximal to the deformity, followed by preparation of the distal femoral metaphysis using intramedullary instrumentation. Trialing should include assessment not only of intra-articular soft tissue balance, and limb and component alignment, but also osteotomy stability. If there is compromised stability of the osteotomy with press fit stem, then an alternative fixation should be sought such as plate fixation or locked intramedullary nailing, with use of an unstemmed femoral component.

Postoperatively, protected weight bearing is allowed until healing has been achieved. Range of motion is encouraged if osteotomy fixation is rigid. Long-term outcome of simultaneous femoral osteotomy and total knee arthroplasty for femoral deformity have been excellent, in terms of durability of the total knee arthroplasty, healing of the osteotomy, and achieving functionability.

References

1. Incavo SJ, Kapadia C, Torney R. Use of an intramedullary nail for correction of femoral deformities combined with total knee arthroplasty: a technical tip. *J Arthrop.* 2007;22:133-135.
2. Lonner JH, Siliski JM, Lotke PA. Simultaneous femoral osteotomy and total knee arthroplasty for treatment of osteoarthritis associated with severe extra-articular deformity. *J Bone Joint Surg.* 2000;82A:342-348.
3. Wang JW, Wang CJ. Total knee arthroplasty for arthritis of the knee with extra-articular deformity. *J Bone Joint Surg.* 2002;84-A:1769-1774.
4. Wolff AM, Hungerford DS, Pepe CL. The effect of extraarticular varus and valgus deformity on total knee arthroplasty. *Clin Orthop.* 1991;271:35-51.

IF A PATIENT HAS A CLEARLY VISIBLE CALCIFIED VESSEL IN THE POSTERIOR ASPECT OF THEIR KNEE ON THE PREOPERATIVE RADIOGRAPH, SHOULD I USE A TOURNIQUET? WHAT ABOUT THE PATIENT WITH A HISTORY OF PRIOR BYPASS GRAFTS?

Raphael C. Y. Hau, MBBS, FRACS
Bassam A. Masri, MD, FRCSC

The use of tourniquets for operative hemostasis in total knee arthroplasty (TKA) remains controversial, and their use, for the most part, depends on surgeon preference. Although the use of a tourniquet provides for a cleaner operative field and may enhance cementation, several potential disadvantages exist including the potential for neurological damage, vascular injury, and compartment syndrome. The use of a tourniquet has also been shown to decrease the skin oxygen level after TKA.

Arterial injuries to the lower limb after TKA, which may be related to tourniquet use can be a devastating complication associated with a substantial risk of lower limb loss and in some cases, mortality. The best strategy to manage this potentially limb- or life-threatening complication is prevention. One group of patients at risk of arterial injuries are those with peripheral vascular disease with or without previous bypass surgery (Figure 4-1). These patients must be identified preoperatively by having a thorough history (searching for evidence of vascular claudication, rest pain, lower extremity ulceration, or a history of prior vascular bypass) and physical examination (such as absent or asymmetric pulses, lack of hair growth, and nail abnormalities).

Figure 4-1. Lateral radiograph of the knee showing calcification of the poplitear artery.

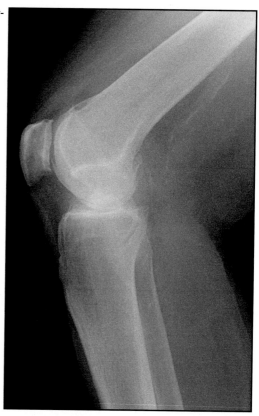

If there is suspicion for vascular insufficiency, the ankle-brachial index (ABI) should be determined by Doppler ultrasound. Patients with clinical symptoms or signs of peripheral vascular disease and an ankle-brachial index (ABI) <0.9 or ABI >1.3 should be assessed by a vascular surgeon preoperatively; patients with an ABI of <0.5 should also have an angiogram preoperatively and be considered for revascularization prior to TKA. A vascular referral should also be made for patients with previous lower limb bypass or angioplasty for the assessment of graft competence. All popliteal aneurysms should be repaired prior to TKA.

At the time of referral, the vascular surgeon should be clearly informed that the patient is awaiting a TKA, and should be asked to provide a written consultation back to the orthopaedic surgeon stating that it is safe for the patient to undergo the procedure knowing that there will be substantial manipulation of the knee at the time of surgery. Caution is necessary in patients with peripheral vascular disease as the tourniquet may cause thrombosis of the popliteal artery secondary to low flow; this represents the most common mechanism of arterial injury following a total knee arthroplasty. Direct mechanical pressure from the tourniquet can also fracture atherosclerotic plaques in the superficial femoral artery leading to distal embolization of plaque fragments.

Calcified vessels tend to have atherosclerotic plaques, and also tend to be less compliant than normal vessels. If the calcified vessels are at the level of the knee or below, and there are normal pedal pulses, it is probably safe to use a tourniquet, if the surgeon so desires. However, if the calcified vessels are more proximally in the thigh (see Figure 4-1), then use of a tourniquet is discouraged as it will be difficult to obtain vascular occlusion secondary to poor compliance of these vessels, unless a very high tourniquet pressure is applied. With an increase in tourniquet pressure, the risk of injuring the atheromas also increases leading to the potential for distal arterial embolization and vascular injury. In patients where a calcified vessel is visualized on the plain radiographs, if palpable pulses are not present then a Doppler ultrasound with ABI is ordered and the patient is sent for evaluation by a vascular surgeon. It is also important to recognize that patients with macrovascular disease oftentimes have concomitant microvascular disease and a tourniquet may further damage the already compromised blood supply to the skin, leading to a higher risk of wound healing problems.

The final group of patients at risk for a vascular injury are those with a history of prior vascular bypass. We obtain a formal consultation from the vascular surgeon who performed the bypass on all of these patients, and we specifically ask whether a tourniquet may be used. Some vascular surgeons recommend that heparin is given prior to tourniquet inflation, and that it is reversed with protamine sulphate at the end of the procedure. With the lack of evidence to conclusively prove that the use of a tourniquet in a knee replacement is associated with concrete advantages, it would be safer to avoid the use of a tourniquet whenever in doubt. Our rule of thumb is if there are any reservation or any concerns about the use of a tourniquet, then it should not be used.

References

1. Smith DE, McGraw RW, Taylor DC, Masri BA. Arterial complications and total knee arthroplasty. *J Am Acad Orthop Surg.* 2001;9:253-257.
2. Clarke MT, Longstaff L, Edwards D, Rushton N. Tourniquet-induced wound hypoxia after total knee replacement. *JBJ. S* 2001;83B:40-44.
3. Graham B, Breault M, McEwen JA, Eng P, McGraw RW. Occlusion of arterial flow in the extremities at subsystolic pressures through the use of wide tourniquet cuffs. *CORR.* 1993;286:257-261.
4. Din R, Geddes T. Skin protection beneath the tourniquet: a prospective randomized trial. *ANZ J Surg.* 2004;74:721-722.

SHOULD MY PATIENTS DONATE BLOOD PRIOR TO SURGERY?

Fred Cushner, MD

If your goal is to maximize your patient's blood levels at the time of discharge as well as minimize their exposure to allogeneic blood transfusions, then the answer is quite clear. Do not have your patients donate autologous prior to a unilateral total knee arthroplasty (TKA).

Donating blood does not result in hypoxia, therefore the patient's own erythropoietin response is not stimulated. We used to think that by donating blood, the patients would return to their predonation hemoglobin (Hb) levels prior to surgery. Multiple studies have shown that this does not occur, however, and patients who have predonated autologous blood arrive for surgery actually with lower Hb levels.[1] We coined the phrase *Orthopaedic Induced Anemia*,[2] and in a recent study documented approximately a 1 g/dl drop in Hb secondary to preoperative autologous donation (PAD). As a result of lower preoperative blood levels, patients are in fact at higher risk for allogeneic transfusion. Not only are PAD donations ineffective at decreasing the risk for allogenic transfusions, they are also costly. Further, the quality of blood (in terms of oxygen carrying capacity) decreases while it sits on a shelf awaiting the indicated surgical procedure.

As a result of numerous studies performed at our institution, we advocate a patient-specific approach that is based on the patient's preoperative Hb level and the procedure to be performed (Figure 5-1).[1,2] Blood management should be no different than other aspects of knee surgery; individualized based on patient needs.

It is well described that the number one factor that predicates a given patient's need for a blood transfusion is their preoperative Hb levels. Patients with lower preoperative Hb levels are at higher risk to receive an allogeneic transfusion than those with higher levels. Specifically, multiple studies have shown that patients with a preoperative Hb of <13 g/dl are at highest risk for allogenic transfusion.

Figure 5-1. Unilateral TKA algorithim for blood management

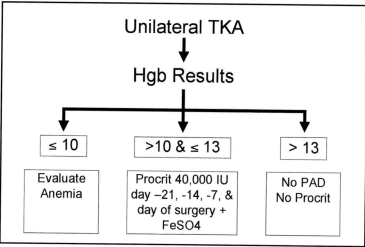

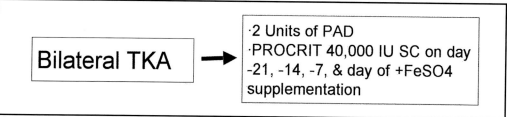

Figure 5-2. Bilateral TKA algorithim for blood management.

Therefore, we screen patients at the time of surgical booking to determine their Hb level. Patients with Hb < 13 g/dl receive a series of weekly epoetin alpha injections (Procrit, Ortho Biotech, Bridgewater, NJ) administered 21, 14, and 7 days prior to surgery with a final dose given on the day of surgery. Patients receive concomitant iron supplementation with an expected rise in Hb of approximately 1.5 g/dl. The success of Procrit injections are well described in the literature and in our experience approximately 1/3 of our patients have a preoperative Hb of <13 and receive Procrit preoperatively.

In a recent series of patients with Hgb > 10 gr/dl and < 13 gr/dl, the answer was quite clear. In these high-risk patients, the group of patients who received Procrit injections, as described earlier, demonstrated a rise in Hb of 1.5 g/dl whereas the PAD group experienced a drop of 1.2 g/dl when their Hb levels were retested on the day of surgery. Thus, the group of patients who received Procrit had a net Hb that was almost 3 g/dl more than patients who donated autologous blood. Further, patients who were treated with Procrit had not only higher Hb levels preoperatively, but also higher Hb levels postoperatively and at the time of discharge.

For bilateral TKA, our protocol is a bit different (Figure 5-2). Patients donate 2 units of blood and also receive Procrit injections to help them "rebound" from the autlogous donation. Utilizing this approach, our allogeneic transfusion rate for bilateral TKA is quite low.[3]

Procrit injections are just part of our blood loss management protocol. We recently reported on the infiltration of the joint capsule with Epinephrine and Lidocaine prior to making our arthrotomy at the time of TKA. In a retrospective review of patients who did and did not have a pericapsular injection utilizing a MIS approach, the mean Hb drop was approximately 1 g/dl less in those who had a pericapsular injection with epinephrine.

Despite overwhelming evidence that a PAD program is suboptimal, many surgeons still recommend to their patients the routine donation of blood prior to primary TKA. A recent survey of members of the American Association of Hip and Knee Surgeons showed that only 7% of members follow a patient-specific approach. Reasons given usually revolve around cost but one must remember that PAD is not without cost. Erythropoetin alpha injections are a prehospital charge and not part of the DRG while PAD donations are costly to the patient as well as the hospital. When costs such as disposal (usually 50 to 75% wastage) as well as the costs of break through allogeneic transfusion are considered, PAD is actually more costly than erythropoietin alpha injections.

These are standard protocols followed at our institution. They are not only efficacious but once explained, easily accepted by our patients.

References

1. Cushner FD, Lee GC, Scuderi GR, Arsht SJ, Scott WN. Blood loss management in high-risk patients undergoing total knee arthroplasty: a comparison of two techniques. *J Knee Surg.* 2006 Oct;17(4):249-253.
2. Cushner FD, Hawes T, Kessler D, Hill K, Scuderi GR. Orthopaedic-induced anemia: the fallacy of autologous donation programs. *Clin Ortho Relat Res.* 2005 Feb;(431): 145-149.
3. Cushner FD, Scott WN, Scuderi GR, Hill K, Insall JN. Blood loss and transfusion rates in bilateral total knee arthroplasty. *Clin Orthop Relat Res.* 2005 Nov;440:170-174.

WHEN DO YOU DO A ONE-STAGE BILATERAL TOTAL KNEE ARTHROPLASTY AS OPPOSED TO STAGING THEM?

Steven Lyons, MD

The decision to do a one-stage bilateral total knee arthoplasty (TKA) versus a staged procedure has been controversial. For the one-stage procedure, choices include either simultaneously with two different surgical teams and two sets of instruments or one surgical team finishing the knees sequentially. Options also exist for the staged approach in regard to timing. Some would consider performing the second surgery while still in the hospital—4 to 7 days later,[1] others 6 weeks, 3 months, or even later. The literature reflects many articles, which both support and refute each methodology and it is the subject of much debate. Conflicting results can be seen for indications, both short- and long-term outcomes as well as perioperative events and complications. All would agree, however, that the decision to perform the TKA should be made on sound evidence based in the literature and hinges on the patients desire, age, and medical comorbidities.

When considering a one-stage bilateral procedure my preference is bilateral simultaneous with the other knee completed by another surgeon in my group at the same time. The only time I sequentially do the knees is if I have to complete both surgeries myself. My experience with bilateral procedures reflects that commonly found in the literature. The patients get both knees done under a shorter anesthetic time, have a lower overall financial burden but spend slightly longer periods in the hospital or rehab and have more complications.[1-4] It is not uncommon to see moderate rates of confusion, delirium, arrhythmia, and the need for blood products postoperatively.[2,4] There is controversy over mortality rates with many studies showing a small increase in the death rate[2] but paradoxically an overall greater life survival.[5]

The one-stage procedure represents a small percentage of TKAs in my practice as many patients have too many health issues to warrant this methodology. I will consider a one-stage bilateral procedure, however, if a healthy motivated patient requests it. In general, I have a rough cut off of 70 years old to stratify the simultaneous versus the staged and restrict the simultaneous procedure to the younger, healthier patient. Medical history plays a critical roll in my decision-making process. Hypertension, diabetes, obesity, and history of cancer are common in my tertiary referral practice and are acknowledged. Any history of cardiovascular disease (such as coronary artery disease or congestive heart failure), respiratory problems (such as emphysema), thromboembolic vents, or stroke is grounds for defaulting to a staged procedure.

Indications that would push me to do a bilateral procedure would be severe bilateral varus or valgus deformities greater than 25 degrees or flexion contractures of 20 degrees or greater in each knee. These types of deformities have been seen to result in less than optimal outcomes if the TKA if completed in a staged fashion. Oftentimes, a recurrent flexion contracture will develop on the side that is operated on first, due to the leg length discrepancy of the operative versus the nonoperative leg. The patient may also be a fall risk due to instability factors in trying to ambulate a "straight leg" alternating with a "malaligned unstable leg." This itself can cause even more problems than the inherent risk of the procedure itself.

When performing simultaneous TKAs all patients are preoperatively cleared and optimized. All receive antibiotics 30 minutes prior to the procedure. The extremities are carefully prepped and draped at the same time and the procedures are started concurrent with each other. Two complete teams are utilized to include one surgeon, one scrub assistant to retract, and one scrub assistant to pass instruments. The same total knee implant system is utilized on each side using an IM rod for alignment of the femur and an extramedullary guide is used for the tibia. The total knee is cemented into place to allow immediate weight bearing and patients are placed on low molecular heparin or Coumadin for thromboembolic prophylaxis. Bilateral CPMs are used and the patients are up walking on the first postoperative day. Discharge usually occurs on postoperative day 4 (as opposed to day 3 for an unilateral TKA) to either home with home health care or a rehabilitation facility. In my experience, a greater percentage of patients require discharge to a rehabilitation facility when a single-stage bilateral procedure is performed secondary to greater postoperative requirements for physical therapy. Ambulation is assisted with a walker for greater stability.

As a tertiary referral surgeon with older patients who oftentimes have significant medical comorbidities, my preference is to stage the TKAs 6 weeks to 3 months apart. In some patients with many medical comorbidities, we further space out the two procedures 6 months to a year apart. This allows the patients to recover from the embolic load from intramedullary fat sustained at the time of operation and also to recover from the surgically induced anemia. Homeostatically it allows them to get back to their "baseline." Also, I feel patients ultimately do better because they can concentrate 100% on rehabbing the operative knee instead of splitting the time they can tolerate physical therapy between the two knees, as is required in bilateral procedures.

In addition to the information presented thus far, when asking patients about their satisfaction with the bilateral procedures, an overwhelming majority would opt for the same approach again.[3] However, I recommend exercising caution in the elderly patient with multiple medical comorbities, specifically cardiovascular.

References

1. Silva CD, Callaghan JJ, Goetz DD, et al. Staggered bilateral total knee arthroplasty performed four to seven days apart during a single hospitalization. *JBJS Am.* 2005;87:508-513.
2. Lane GJ, Hozack WJ, Shah S, et al. Simultaneous bilateral versus unilateral total knee arthroplasty: outcomes analysis. *Clin Orthop.* 1997;12:106-112.
3. Leonard L, Williamson DM, Ivory JP, Jennison C. An evaluation of the safety and efficacy of simultaneous bilateral total knee arthroplasty. *J Arthroplasty.* 2003;8:972-978.
4. Lynch NM, Trousdale RT, Ilstrup DM. Complications after concomitant bilateral total knee arthroplasty in elderly patients. *Mayo Clin Proc.* 1997;72:799.
5. Ritter MA, Harty LD, Davis KE, Meding JB, Berend M. Simultaneous bilateral, staged bilateral, and unilateral total knee arthroplasty. A survival analysis. *JBJS Am.* 2003;85:1532-1537.

SHOULD THE PATELLA BE ROUTINELY RESURFACED AT THE TIME OF TOTAL KNEE ARTHOPLASTY?

Javad Parvizi, MD, FRCS
Feridon Jaberi, MD

I personally always resurface the patella during primary total knee arthroplasty (TKA). A meta-analysis found that the incidence of anterior knee pain was 15.5% in patients with patellar resurfacing and twice as much at 30.3% for those without resurfacing. The relative risk of anterior knee pain was found to be 0.35 in the same meta-analysis and, thus, for every 7 patients undergoing TKA with patellar resurfacing, one instance of clinically important anterior knee pain may be avoided.

However, I realize there are surgeons who "never" resurface the patella or "selectively" resurface the patella. To give you a balanced view I think that the patella should be resurfaced in patients with anterior knee pain and evidence of "severe" degenerative disease in the patellofemoral joint. Isolated patellofemoral (PF) arthritis is another indication for resurfacing of the patella. Most, surgeons would also resurface the patella in patients with inflammatory arthritis such as rheumatoid arthritis.

I resurface the patella because of three main reasons:

1. I cannot predict which patients will have anterior knee pain after TKA. If I leave the patella unresurfaced and the patient presents with anterior knee pain postoperatively, then I would "blame" the unresurfaced patella for this problem, realizing that there are patients with resurfaced patella who have anterior knee pain as well.

2. My eyes are not good at judging the thickness or the quality of the patellar cartilage. Hence, I cannot predict what will happen to the patellar cartilage over the lifetime of the TKA.

3. I want to minimize the chances of reoperating on patients. Based on a published meta-analysis the incidence of secondary resurfacing of the patella is around 8%.

The question is: Why doesn't every surgeon resurface the patella? Advocates of nonresurfacing cite a higher incidence of patellofemoral complications such as avascular necrosis and fracture as reasons to not resurface the patella in every patient.[1,2] They also argue that the biomechanics of the knee in general, and the quadriceps mechanism in particular, may be affected by patellar resurfacing. In addition, patellar resurfacing adds operative time, is more expensive (secondary to the cost of patellar component), "gets rid" of good cartilage in some patients, and may lead to early wear and failure of the entire TKA when suboptimal patellar prosthesis are used.

I would argue, however, that the incidence of patellar fracture and avasular necrosis is very low when the patella is resurfaced. If one is careful during resurfacing (see later for explanations) then patellar complications should be minimal. Further, suboptimal patellar prostheses such as metal-backed and central peg patellae designs (that lead to higher incidence of avascular necrosis) have been discontinued.

Opponents of resurfacing would also argue that, with the introduction of better-designed knee prostheses (such as those with deeper trochlear groove and a thinner anterior femoral flange), the incidence of anterior knee pain or problems related to unresurfaced patella has decreased. In other words, they believe that the performance of TKA is more dependent on the design of the knee as opposed to whether the patella was resurfaced or not. I would agree with this concept fully.

In my opinion there may be three situations during which strong argument for nonresurfacing of patella is offered:

1. Very young and active patients in whom preservation of bone stock in patella is advantageous.
2. Very obese patients who may place undue forces on their resurfaced patella.
3. Patients in whom native patella is very thin (<12 mm).

How to Resurface

If the patella is to be resurfaced, there are some surgical pointers that may help avoid complications. During the bone cut I irrigate the patella in order to minimize heat necrosis. I do not dissect out the entire fat pad and only remove a small portion to assist visualization. I avoid skeletonizing the patellar tendon. In addition, I take necessary steps to ensure that the knee components are well positioned to avoid lateral retinacular release. All of the aforementioned should help minimize disruption of blood supply to the patella.

To avoid affecting the lever arm of the quadriceps mechanism, I always measure the thickness of the patella and attempt to restore the same patellar height, or perhaps 1 mm less, with the resurfacing. Excessive patellar thickness can cause maltracking due to its effect on overall shortening of the quadriceps excursion. I am also extremely careful to produce a symmetrical cut that is in line with the anterior cortex. The most common mistake is the failure to define the medial chondro-osseous junction, so the patellar cut is shallower on the medial side. Following completion of the cut I use a patellar caliper that allows measurement of all four quadrants. Feeling the patella for thickness and symmetry is also very useful. I also always check for dynamic stability of the patella to ensure appropriate tracking and congruency with the trochlear groove.

Bibliography

Barrack RL, Wolfe MW, Waldman DA, Milicic M, Bertot AJ, Myers L. Surfacing of the patella in total knee arthroplasty. A prospective, randomized, double blind study. *J Bone Joint Surg Am.* 1997;79(8):1121-1131.

Burnett RS, Haydon CM, Rorabeck CH, Bourne RB. Patella resurfacing versus nonresurfacing in total knee arthroplasty: results of a randomized controlled clinical trial at a minimum of 10 years' follow-up. *Clin Orthop Relat Res.* 2004;(428):12-25.

Parvizi J, Rapuri VR, Saleh KJ, Kuskowski MA, Sharkey PF, Mont MA. Failure to resurface the patella during total knee arthroplasty may result in more knee pain and secondary surgery. *Clin Orthop Relat Res.* 2005;438:191-196.

I HAVE A PATIENT WHO IS VERY CONCERNED ABOUT THEIR RANGE OF MOTION. SHOULD I USE A HIGH FLEX TYPE COMPONENT?

Giles R. Scuderi, MD

Postoperative range of motion (ROM) following total knee arthroplasty (TKA) is influenced by patient-related factors, surgical technique, and implant design. Additional factors influencing the postoperative ROM include previous surgery, which may induce arthrofibrosis, as well as the severity of the arthritic process. However, it has been well established that the preoperative ROM is the strongest indicator of postoperative ROM.[1]

Some patients have both high flexibility and the desire to perform deep flexion activities. This is especially true in ethnic populations that require flexion >120 degrees for social, religious, or working activities; a successful result in this patient group demands not only relief of pain but also the restoration of ROM. It has been reported that walking and climbing slopes requires <90 degrees of flexion; climbing stairs and arising from a chair 90 to 120 degrees of flexion; getting in and out of a bath tub 135 degrees of flexion; kneeling, squatting and sitting cross-legged requires 110 to 165 degrees; and activities like golf, meditation, yoga, and gardening often require flexion >150 degrees.

Preoperative evaluation is useful in identifying patients that will achieve high flexion postoperatively. The patient should express a need for high flexion activities, have a preoperative ROM >120 degrees, a stable knee, and not be obese (the thigh and calf soft tissues can impinge before the knee flexes to 90 degrees in heavy individuals). It must be stressed preoperatively to the patient that in order for high flexion to be achieved, they must be an active participant in their postoperative rehabilitation program.

Surgical technique also impacts ROM.[2] The principle of balanced gaps must be followed. It is imperative to resect the tibia at the right level with an appropriate posterior slope and place the tibial component in the correct rotation. Femoral component sizing is similarly important, with restoration of both the anterior-posterior dimension and posterior condylar offset being critical. Bellemans has shown that restoring the femoral posterior condylar offset impacts the degree of knee flexion.[3] It is important to remove posterior femoral osteophytes and release the posterior capsule in order to reestablish the posterior recess. Failure to do this will result in impingement of the posterior aspect of the tibia on the posterior aspect of the femur. This mechanical impingement has also been observed with PCL retaining knee prostheses when there is abnormal kinematics and the paradoxical anterior femoral translation during flexion.[2]

Current high flexion prostheses are specifically designed for safe flexion to 155 degrees. While there are cruciate retaining high flexion knee prostheses available, it is preferable to design a high flexion knee with a posterior cruciate substituting articulation.[2] Posterior stabilized knees have shown predictable femoral rollback throughout flexion by the interaction of the femoral cam and tibial spine mechanism. In order to maintain stability as the knee flexes, it is important that as the femoral cam engages the tibial spine it moves down the tibial spine. This creates a higher jump distance, imparts stability in deep flexion, and reduces the stress on the tibial spine. In designing the frontal geometry, a conforming round on round articulation increases the contact area and reduces contact stresses on the polyethylene. In designing the sagittal geometry of the femoral component, there is a distinct advantage to multiple radii. Maximum conformity can be achieved in full extension and early flexion during gait. A decreasing sagittal radius permits improved flexion without the kinematic conflict of conformity and constraint with a single radius design. Finally, as the knee comes into full flexion, in order to avoid edge loading, the posterior condyles are extended, providing a larger contact area with the tibial articular surfaces. A flexion-friendly patellofemoral articulation is also required with a trochlea deep enough to reduce the stresses on the patella and accommodate high flexion. To reduce patella and patella tendon impingement in deep flexion, the anterior lip of the tibial polyethylene articular surface should be recessed.

Recent clinical studies have revealed that high flexion is achievable. Huang et al. reported an average postoperative ROM of 138 degrees at 2-year follow-up with the LPS Flex Prosthesis (Zimmer, Warsaw, IN); a 25% increase in ROM compared to an average preoperative ROM of 110 degrees.[4] Similarly, Kim et al reported an average ROM of 139 degrees with the same prosthesis at the same follow-up interval.[5] Similar ROM can be achieved with a standard prosthesis, but the LPS Flex prosthesis better restores the posterior condylar offset and is specifically designed for safe flexion beyond 125 degrees. Argenson et al. have shown that patients implanted with a high flexion design had kinematic patterns that were similar to the healthy knee.[6] The restoration of normal femorotibial kinematics with high weight bearing ROM may be related to the specific design features of the high flexion prosthesis. The in vivo kinematic evaluation of patients with the LPS Flex prosthesis has demonstrated remarkable femorotibial kinematics with a high incidence of posterior femoral rollback, minimal condylar lift-off, and excellent ROM under weight bearing conditions.[2]

High flexion TKA requires appropriate preoperative evaluation and patient education, adherence to the surgical techniques mentioned earlier, and an implant that is designed to safely accommodate flexion to 155 degrees. Following these recommendations for high flexion TKA, the patient's and surgeon's expectations will be matched and satisfied.

References

1. Ritter MA, Harty LD, Davis KE, Meding JB, Berend M. Predicting range of motion after total knee arthroplasty: Clustering, log-linear regression and regression tree analysis. *JBJS*. 2003;85A:1278-1285.
2. Argenson JN, Scuderi GR, Komistek RD, Scott WN, Kelly MA, Aubaniac JM. In vivo kinematic evaluation and design considerations related to high flexion in total knee arthroplasty. *J Biomechanics*. 2005;38:277-284.
3. Bellemans J, Banks S, Victor J, Vandenneucker H, Moemans A. A fluoroscopic analysis of the kinematics of deep flexion in total knee arthroplasty. Influence of posterior condylar offset. *J Bone Joint Surg*. 2002;84B:50-53.
4. Huang HT, Su JY, Wang GJ. The early results of high flexion total knee arthroplasty. A minimum of 2 years follow-up. *J Arthroplasty*. 2005;20(5):674-679.
5. Kim YH, Sohn KS, Kim SHL. Range of motion of standard and high flexion posterior stabilized total knee prostheses. *J Bone Joint Surg*. 2005;87A:1470-1475.
6. Argenson JN, Komistek RD, Mahfouz M, Walker SA, Aubaniac JM, Dennis DA. A high flexion total knee arthroplasty design replicates healthy knee motion. *Clin Orthop*. 2004;428:174-179.

I HAVE A 43-YEAR-OLD MALE WHO NEEDS A TOTAL KNEE: SHOULD I USE HIGHLY CROSS-LINKED POLYETHYLENE AS A BEARING SURFACE?

Markus A. Wimmer, PhD
Joshua J. Jacobs, MD

From a scientific view point this question cannot be answered with a clear "yes" or "no." Presently, there is no clinical data with a sufficient follow-up period allowing us to address such a question in a direct way. Therefore, in the following paragraphs we will provide a summary of the pros and cons of cross-linked polyethylenes for total knee arthroplasty—based mostly on in vitro test results. Time will tell whether those results accurately reflect the long-term in vivo behavior of highly cross-linked polyethylene.

Ultra-high molecular weight polyethylene (UHMWPE) has always been the norm as a bearing surface in total knee replacement. For total hip arthroplasty, there has recently been a push toward the use of highly cross-linked UHMWPE for the high-demand patient. This is due to the fact that this patient population experiences a relatively high prevalence of osteolysis with conventional bearing couplings (cobalt chrome head on a conventional polyethylene socket liner) at intermediate to long-term follow-up. It is widely accepted that osteolysis is in large part the host's response to the generation of a large volume of polyethylene wear debris, which leads to particle phagocytosis, the secretion of pro-inflammatory cytokines, and osteoclastogenic factors that ultimately result in increased bone resorption and decreased bone formation in the periprosthetic bone.[1] Lower wear of alternative bearing surfaces may diminish this problem in the hip and short- to intermediate-term results are promising. In particular, randomized controlled trials using highly cross-linked polyethylene in the hip suggests a substantial reduction in clinical wear rates.[2] It is reasonable to presume that this reduction in wear rates will be translated into improved survivorships of total hip arthroplasties in the high-demand patient.

Figure 9-1. Anteroposterior radiograph of a cementless total knee replacement reconstruction demonstrating extensive proximal tibial osteolysis in association with adjuvant screw fixation.

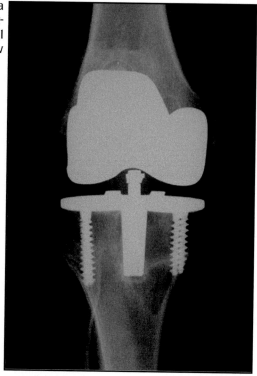

Is this state of affairs in the hip joint transferable to the knee joint? Osteolysis is seen in total knee replacement,[3] although not to the same extent as in total hip arthroplasty. It is clear that osteolysis has been reported as a clinical problem about the knee, however this seems to be design specific and in some series related to the method of fixation. High prevalences of osteolysis were noted in certain systems that were susceptible to accelerated polyethylene wear, either on the articular or the back surface. In some systems osteolysis was associated with the screws used in cementless tibial component fixation (Figure 9-1).

In most total knee designs, the tibiofemoral articulation undergoes a rolling/sliding motion as opposed to pure sliding in the hip joint. As a result, surface fatigue becomes the dominant wear mechanism, and adhesion, the prevailing wear mechanism in the artificial hip, becomes secondary.[4] This is reflected in the particle size where it is known that the particulate debris generated from polyethylene bearings surfaces in total knee arthroplasty tends to be larger and thus will tend to be less bioreactive. Furthermore, the capacity of the synovial space in the knee is typically greater than the hip. Finally, there are differential access pathways in the hip and the knee that may lead to a differential prevalence of osteolysis. In general, with a number of contemporary implant systems, the occurrence of osteolysis at 10 to 15 years postoperative is typically less than what is seen in a number of hip arthroplasty systems.

Backside wear of the polyethylene undersurface has been identified as a major particle source.[5] During cyclic loading of the implant, the polyethylene insert undergoes fretting wear against the tibial metal tray and generates particles in the submicron range. Dependent on the locking mechanism and surface finish, the volume of material removed can be substantial and may be sufficient to induce osteolysis. Similarly, rotating platform knees produce small particles due to their reciprocating sliding wear mode at the undersurface of the insert. Therefore, for selected designs—and for the high-demand patient—there may be a rationale to use highly cross-linked UHMWPE.

It is well known that highly cross-linked polyethylene materials, while having improved wear characteristics, do have reduced fracture toughness as well as reduced fatigue crack propagation resistance.[6] This is a substantial tradeoff since—as mentioned earlier—surface fatigue has to be expected as the prevalent wear mechanism during rolling/sliding in total knee replacement. The articulating surfaces in the knee may therefore be more prone to fracture than the hip. In addition, there are other geometric features on the articulating surfaces in the knee that may be prone to fracture as well (posts, cutouts, dovetails, etc). Hence, new material developments must take this into account. In fact, many manufacturers use a different formulation for the highly cross-linked materials in the knee as compared to the hip; lower radiation doses would be used to minimize the decrement in fracture toughness.

In conclusion, in total knee arthroplasty fatigue and fracture resistance of UHMWPE are as important as wear properties. Highly cross-linked polyethylenes are an option for the young and active high-demand patient as long as sufficient fracture and fatigue resistance can be guaranteed. Given that we are seeking survivorships in excess of two decades, for which we currently have very little clinical information on the current generation of "conventional" polyethylene, there may indeed be a place for a more wear resistant polyethylene. Current in vitro knee simulations are promising in terms of the ability of this material to reduce wear.

References

1. Jacobs JJ, Roebuck KA, Archibeck M, Hallab NJ, Glant TT. Osteolysis: basic science. *Clin Orthop Relat Res.* 2001;393:71-77.
2. Digas G, Karrholm J, Thanner J, Malchau H, Herberts P. Highly cross-linked polyethylene in total hip arthroplasty: randomized evaluation of penetration rate in cemented and uncemented sockets using radiostereometric analysis. *Clin Orthop Relat Res.* 2004;429:6-16.
3. Naudie DD, Ammeen DJ, Engh GA, Rorabeck CH. Wear and osteolysis around total knee arthroplasty. *J Am Acad Orthop Surg.* 2007;1:53-64.
4. Wimmer MA, Andriacchi, TP. Chapter 9: Human motion and its relevance to wear and failure in total knee arthroplasty. In: Shanbhag A, Rubash HE, Jacobs JJ, eds., *Joint Replacement and Bone Resorption: Pathology, Biomaterials, and Clinical Practice.* New York, NY: Taylor & Francis; 2006:171-210.
5. Conditt MA, Thompson MT, Usrey MM, Ismaily SK, Noble PC. Backside wear of polyethylene tibial inserts: mechanism and magnitude of material loss. *J Bone Joint Surg [Am].* 2005;87:326-331.
6. Puertolas JA, Medel FJ, Cegonino J, Gomez-Barrena E, Rios R. Influence of the remelting process on the fatigue behavior of electron beam irradiated UHMWPE. *J Biomed Mater Res [B].* 2006;76:346-353.

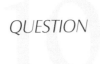
I Think My Patient May Have a Charcot (Neuropathic) Knee. Is This a Contraindication to Total Knee Arthroplasty?

R. Michael Meneghini, MD
Jeffery L. Pierson, MD

Neuropathic arthropathy of the knee, or what is commonly referred to as a *Charcot knee*, represents a unique pathologic condition with an unknown etiology. It is thought to result from diminished proprioception, which renders the knee susceptible to repetitive microtrauma and destruction due to the lack of protective sensation. Charcot arthropathy is associated with a number of diseases that affect the nervous system, including diabetes mellitus, tertiary syphilis (tabes dorsalis), and familial sensorimotor deficit, yet a certain number are considered idiopathic in etiology.

Patients typically present with a warm, swollen, and a frequently unstable knee. The joint is usually relatively painless; however, up to 50% of neuropathic joints can be painful and clinical presentation can be confused with septic arthritis. Patients suspected of having a Charcot knee should be referred for complete medical and neurological evaluation to determine if a treatable etiology exists. Serologic testing should include testing for syphilis, glucose tolerance, and a complete blood count to include evaluation for vitamin B_{12} or thiamine deficiency, as well as sedimentation rate and C-reactive protein to evaluate for a potential infection. In some cases, nerve conduction studies can be helpful for establishing the diagnosis of neuropathic arthropathy. Radiographic evaluation should include anterioposterior, lateral, merchant, and long mechanical axis views of the affected knee and extremity. Characteristic radiographic features include joint destruction, osseous fragmentation involving the femur and tibia, subluxation, periarticular bone formation, and progressive angular deformity in the end-stage of the disease (Figure 10-1).

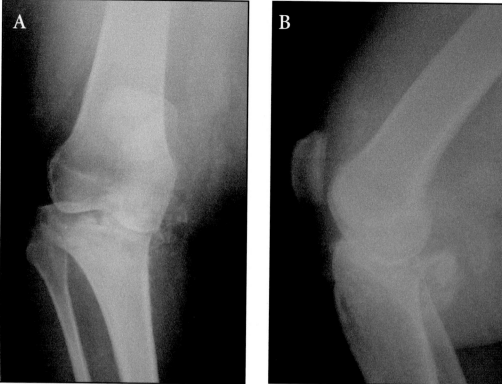

Figure 10-1. Preoperative AP (A) and lateral (B) radiographs of a knee with neuropathic (Charcot) arthropathy demonstrating the characteristic bone destruction, periarticular bone formation, subluxation, and progressive varus deformity.

Previously, a Charcot knee was considered a contraindication to total knee replacement; however, with improved implant designs and an awareness of the technical and surgical nuances involved with these patients, total knee arthroplasty is currently an acceptable treatment that can reliably restore and improve knee function. Careful and thorough surgical planning must be performed to adequately address the multitude of pitfalls that may be encountered when performing knee replacement in these difficult patients. Surgical exposure can be challenging and must be undertaken carefully to avoid the numerous potential complications such as medial collateral ligament or patellar tendon avulsion. Extensor malalignment is frequently observed and may require lateral retinacular release and/or tibial tubercle transfer or advancement.[1] Ligamentous instability requires the use of at minimum a posterior cruciate substituting prosthesis. In many cases, a constrained condylar prosthesis is required to restore knee stability. As such, stem extensions are frequently required to address the increased articular constraint and to provide supplemental fixation for the frequently encountered osseous defects. Fragmentation of bone and severe defects frequently are present and may require the use of metal block augmentation or bone grafts (Figure 10-2).

Historically, results of total knee arthroplasty in patients with neuropathic arthropathy have been suboptimal. In an early report of 24 knees undergoing total knee replacement, the authors report a high complication rate and an alarming 50% failure rate by 2 years fol-

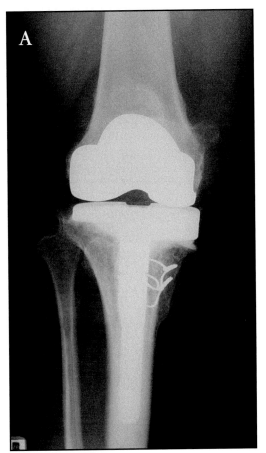 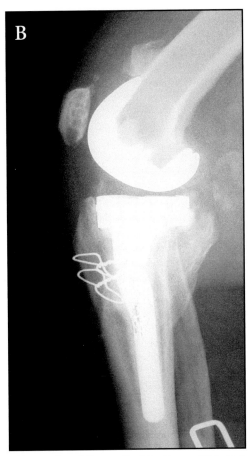

Figure 10-2. Postoperative AP (A) and lateral (B) radiographs of the patient in Figure 10-1 at 1 year postoperatively. A long-stem tibial component and metal augmentation was required to address the osseous defect and a tibial tubercle osteotomy was required to facilitate the difficult surgical exposure.

low-up. However, the results of that study were markedly confounded by numerous knees with poor prosthetic design and there was an 82% success rate of condylar prosthesis at 4 years.[2] A recent report of 19 total knee replacements in 10 patients with neurosyphylitic Charcot arthropathy documented a 53% satisfactory outcome at minimum 5 years using a constrained condylar design. Three knees were revised for aseptic loosening and despite the high complication rate, the authors concluded that Charcot arthropathy was not an absolute contraindication for total knee replacement.[3] In the most recent study, Parvizi et al reported on 40 total knee replacements of a modern condylar design performed for the diagnosis of Charcot knee.[1] The authors documented the need for metal augmentation, bone grafting, and long stems for bony defects and ligamentous instability. At a mean 7.9 years follow-up, there was a significant improvement in pain and function in this patient group, despite 6 reoperations for periprosthetic fracture, aseptic loosening, instability, and deep infection. The authors recommend TKR as an appropriate treatment for neuropathic arthropathy with an understanding that the procedure requires surgical skills, implants, and methods that are typically used in complex revision arthroplasty.[1]

References

1. Parvizi J, Marrs J, Morrey, BF. Total knee arthroplasty for neuropathic (Charcot) joints. *Clin Orthop Relat Res.* 2003;(416):145-150.
2. Doherty WP, Rand JA, Bryan RS. Total knee arthroplasty in neuropathic arthropathy. In: *Total Knee Arthroplasty of the Knee: Proceedings of the Knee Society, 1985–1986.* Rockville, MD: Aspen Publishers; 1987:279-285.
3. Kim, YH, Kim JS, Oh SW. Total knee arthroplasty in neuropathic arthropathy. *J Bone Joint Surg Br.* 2002; 84(2):216-219.

I Am Considering Implementing a Teaching Class Prior to Surgery for My Patients. Is This Beneficial? What Topics Should Be Covered?

Regina Barden, RN, BSN
Kim Chandler, RN, BSN

Patient education plays a crucial role in optimizing a patient's surgical experience and outcome. The communication process between a physician and the patient to discuss the patient's diagnosis and treatment options is not only an ethical obligation but also a legal requirement.[1] Studies have shown that preoperative education helps to alleviate patient fears, and decreases anxiety, length of stay, and postsurgical pain. Education also improves patient satisfaction.[2] Once a patient has been informed that they are a candidate for knee replacement surgery, it is the responsibility of the surgeon and his/her staff to provide the necessary education. The purpose of educating patients is to provide information about the surgical intervention and to help them develop realistic expectations. This will allow them to make an educated, informed decision about consenting to surgery. We have used preoperative teaching in our practice for more than 20 years and feel it is a cornerstone of quality care.

Studies have show that retention of medical information given in a verbal session with a health care provider may be less than 50%.[3] We believe that repetition of teaching materials and reinforcement of important concepts can help patients gain a better understanding of the material. The combination of verbal instruction and written materials along with Web site–based programs is an approach that we have found to be very effective for patients and caregivers. These are all acceptable methods to educate patients, but one has to remember that there are barriers that affect how much information a patient retains with any one method. Barriers to learning may include: education level, illiteracy, language differences, hearing or visual impairment, psychological and physical disabilities, and lack of access to electronic equipment to view teaching programs.

Verbal instruction can be customized to patients' needs through an individual or group approach. Verbal instruction promotes a more personal interactive learning approach. Giving patients the opportunity to have their questions answered during a session aids in the understanding of the material. In our experience, a one on one session may be more appropriate for individuals with special physical and psychosocial needs and patients that may not tolerate a class setting.

Classes for preoperative teaching can be a very effective way to deliver information to several patients at one time, undergoing the same procedure. Family members or significant others are encouraged to come with the patient to gain a better understanding of how to support the patient. We encourage our patients to review supplemental written education materials before coming to class.

Classes can be taught by an individual representative of the health care team or as a multidisciplinary approach. This may be hospital based or developed through private practices. It is important that whoever leads these sessions is a dedicated, enthusiastic person. Our patients are divided into surgeon-specific classes. This allows for discussion of individual protocols. We feel that a multidisciplinary approach including the surgeon's clinical nurse or physician assistant along with a physical therapist, hospital nurse, and social worker provides a more comprehensive education. Patients have various knowledge levels, so be sure to teach at an understandable level. You want to make all patients feel welcome. Group format provides an opportunity for patients and significant others to network. Listening to other people's questions and answers can help alleviate fears and concerns about surgery. An established multidisciplinary education program showed that an interactive program with immediate feedback was a positive experience for patients.[4]

The class size and length of session are important considerations. Allow enough room for patients to bring a significant other. It is important that they are taught in a comfortable environment with limited distractions. We feel that a class size of 12 to 15 patients along with significant others is a manageable group. Class length of approximately 1 hour seems to keep patients' attention. Patients should be assigned a specific class time by the office staff to avoid overattendance. The number of classes taught is dependent on the number of surgeries scheduled. We recommend at least one class each week. Primary and revision surgery can be combined although this is not ideal. Coordinating medical appointments in conjunction with the class makes it more convenient for patients. Offering evening and weekend classes is an option for working patients.

Content of teaching session:
* Anatomy of knee/disease process
* Overview of surgical procedure
* Risks and benefits of surgery
* Hospital stay
* Equipment used
* Pain management protocol
* Discharge planning
* Rehabilitation/physical therapy
* Recovery period/restrictions

At the end of the class, if the patient has no further questions, have them sign their informed consent along with an information form that states they understand the risks of surgery. This can be witnessed by the class instructor. A periodic survey at the end of the session is helpful to assess effectiveness and the need for content changes.

It is up to the surgeon to determine how his/her patients will be educated. Whatever method is used, it should be a mandatory part of your practice. Our goal of preoperative education is to inform patients about a procedure, answer all questions, and ultimately decrease a patient's anxiety about surgery. Customized or standardized written information, access to teaching Web sites, and videos are important for the patient and families to use as reference materials. The more a person sees or hears the information, the greater the chance they will retain the material. To help protect yourself in litigation, it is important that the education and communication process with the patient be documented in the patient's chart.

References

1. AMA (Legal Issues) Informed Consent. Retrieved December 29, 2006, from http://www.ama-assn.org/ama/pub/category/print/4608.html.
2. Suldham C. A review of the impact of preoperative education on recovery from surgery. *Inter J Nursing Studies*. 1999;36(2):171-177.
3. Geier KA. Improving outcomes in elective orthopaedic surgery: a guide for nurses and total joint arthroplasty patients. *Orthopaedic Nursing* (supplement). 2000;19:3-34.
4. Prouty A, Cooper M, Thomas P, Christiensen J, Strong C, Bowie L, Oermann M. Multidisciplinary patient education for total joint replacement surgery patients. *Orthopaedic Nursing*. 2006; 25(4):257-261.

SECTION II

INTRAOPERATIVE QUESTIONS

IF A PATIENT HAS HAD PRIOR SURGERY, HOW DO I DECIDE WHERE TO MAKE THE SKIN INCISION?

Brett Levine, MD, MS

Introduction

Choosing a skin incision for a total knee arthroplasty (TKA) following previous open surgical procedures can be challenging. In order to avoid skin necrosis and wound complications, it is paramount that these prior surgical incisions not be ignored.

Anatomy

The majority of the blood supply to the skin arises medially from the saphenous and descending geniculate arteries. These vessels supply the deep perforators that pierce the overlying fascia, forming a network of vessels superficial to the fascial layer (Figure 12-1).[1] Blood vessels from the superficial plexus extend through the subcutaneous tissues and link with the dermal plexus. This plexus, in turn, supplies the dermal and epidermal layers of skin. There is minimal communication between these ascending vessels in the subcutaneous fat and, thus, I always make full-thickness flaps when performing soft-tissue dissection during TKA.[1] Extensive dissection superficial to the fascia will disrupt this precarious blood supply and compromise wound healing. Similarly, I never make parallel incisions in close proximity to one another as they can diminish the circulation to the surrounding skin. Finally, it is important not to confuse the blood supply of the patella with that of the skin, as there is little communication between the two structures.[1]

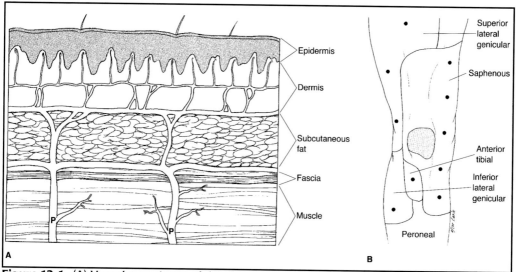

Figure 12-1. (A) Vascular anatomy of the skin of the thigh. (B) Areas supplied by the deep vessels of the knee. ©1998 American Academy of Orthopaedic Surgeons. Reprinted from the *J Am Acad Orthopaedic Surgeons*. 1998;6(1):55-64 with permission.

Choosing Your Skin Incision

In 1988, Johnson reported that the three most important factors for wound healing were: (1) orientation of the incision to skin cleavage lines; (2) skin tension during healing; and (3) viability of the skin edges.[2] These factors may be divided into pre-, intra-, and postoperative issues that if evaluated thoroughly can lead to choosing and executing an optimal incision.

As with most decisions in medicine, I start with a detailed history to identify medical comorbidities that may predispose to wound complications including immunosuppression, malnutrition, steroid use, rheumatoid arthritis, peripheral vascular disease, diabetes, tobacco use, renal insufficiency, prior radiation, and a history of delayed wound healing. If any of these factors are present, I send the patient for a preoperative consultation with a plastic surgeon (to evaluate the patient for a tissue expander or flap coverage) and/or a vascular surgeon (to determine if a revascularization procedure is needed).[3] On physical exam, I carefully assess the mobility of the skin; scars that are immobile and adherent to the underlying deep tissues are more likely to be problematic and less likely to heal uneventfully. Further, I do not hesitate to send patients for preoperative transcutaneous oxygen pressure measurements (TcPO$_2$) as it has been shown that wounds with a TcPO$_2$ of less than 20 torr are unlikely to heal, whereas those greater than 40 torr generally heal well.[4]

Intraoperatively, I mark all prior incisions and if necessary retain the services of a plastic surgeon to assist with choosing the optimal incision, especially if there is a high likelihood of needing a flap or skin graft for wound coverage. If previous longitudinal incisions exist, I incorporate the lateral-most incision that is likely to afford adequate exposure. Due to the medially based blood supply, I would rather elevate a full-thickness medial flap than a lateral one. If unable to incorporate a lateral incision, then maintaining

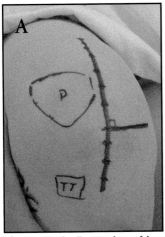 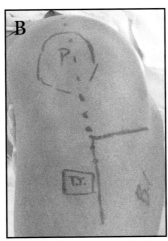 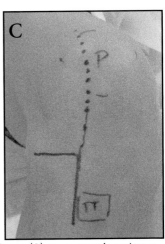

Figure 12-2. Examples of how to handle previous surgical incisions: (A) open meniscectomy—the old incision is crossed in a perpendicular fashion, (B) high tibial osteotomy—the vertical limb of the incision is continued proximally, (C) open reduction and internal fixation of a lateral tibial plateau fracture—the vertical limb of the incision is extended proximally and either a lateral parapatellar arthrotomy or a large medial full-thickness flap maybe elevated to approach the knee.

the widest possible skin bridge between the incisions, without compromising exposure, is the best option. When prior transverse incisions are present, it is safe to cross these incisions in a perpendicular manner, while avoiding intersecting angles less than 60 degrees.[1] If possible, the distal extent of the skin incision should be directed medial to the tibial tubercle so as to avoid injury to the underlying patellar tendon. I find that extension of previous incisions is helpful in identifying normal tissue planes and facilitating exposure and maintenance of full-thickness skin flaps. It is generally safe to ignore short medial or lateral incisions (ie, arthroscopy portals), however, it wise to be more cautious when dealing with wide scars with minimal subcutaneous tissue (indicative of a probable underlying dermal plexus injury).[1] Figure 12-2 shows some examples of how I handled previous skin incisions.

In the postoperative setting, Johnson has shown that peri-incisional $TcPO_2$ levels decrease for the first 2 to 3 days after surgery with the lateral edge of the incision being more hypoxic.[5] It has also been suggested that skin tension may exacerbate this hypoxia and inhibit early angiogenesis and migration of fibroblasts and macrophages necessary for wound healing.[2,6] Therefore, if there is any question of wound healing, early immobilization or delayed mobilization (limit motion to 60 degrees of flexion) for the first 7 to 10 days is my treatment protocol.

Conclusion

The most important rules to follow in choosing your TKA incision are:
1. Respect the medially based vascular anatomy of the skin.
2. Incorporate previous incisions.

3. Transverse incisions may be crossed perpendicular to the scar.

4. If longitudinal incisions exist, choose the lateral most incision that affords appropriate exposure.

5. Consult plastic and/or vascular surgeons preoperatively.

6. Maintain full-thickness flaps (avoid dissection superficial to the deep fascia).

7. In tenuous wounds, avoid aggressive early range of motion.

References

1. Younger AS, Duncan CP, Masri BA. Surgical exposures in revision total knee arthroplasty. *J Am Acad Orthop Surg.* 1998;6(1):55-64.
2. Johnson DP. Midline or parapatellar incision for knee arthroplasty. A comparative study of wound viability. *J Bone Joint Surg Br.* 1988;70(4):656-658.
3. Ries MD. Skin necrosis after total knee arthroplasty. *J Arthroplasty.* 2002;17(4)(Suppl 1):74-77.
4. Bacharach JM, Rooke TW, Osmundson PJ, Gloviczki P. Predictive value of transcutaneous oxygen pressure and amputation success by use of supine and elevation measurements. *J Vasc Surg.* 1992;15(3):558-563.
5. Johnson DP. The effect of continuous passive motion on wound-healing and joint mobility after knee arthroplasty. *J Bone Joint Surg Am.* 1990;72(3):421-426.
6. Yashar AA, Venn-Watson E, Welsh T, Colwell CW, Jr., Lotke P. Continuous passive motion with accelerated flexion after total knee arthroplasty. *Clin Orthop Relat Res.* 1997;(345):38-43.

IF I AM DOING A TOTAL KNEE ARTHROPLASTY AND THE PATELLA DOES NOT SEEM TO TRACK WELL, WHAT SHOULD I DO?

Richard A. Berger, MD

We have been taught to concentrate on balancing the flexion and the extension gaps while obtaining balanced varus/valgus stability. Thus, the patellar arthroplasty has, up until recently, really been an afterthought. Therefore, it is not surprising that patellofemoral complications are the most common complications in total knee arthroplasty.[1] All of these late problems manifest themselves intraoperatively as patella maltracking or subluxation. This condition must be addressed when discovered intraoperatively.

Releasing the Lateral Retinaculum Just Doesn't Work

It is easy to think that patellofemoral maltracking is secondary to a tight lateral retinaculum and, therefore, a lateral retinacular release will resolve the problem. However, a lateral retinacular release rarely improves the problem, since the retinaculum is not the problem; it is really only a symptom that we have, in some way, altered the patellofemoral articulation.

Occasionally, such as in a knee with a valgus deformity, real lateral retinacular tightness is identified preoperatively. On these occasions, a lateral retinacular release is appropriate. However, in the majority of knees the patella tracks quite well prior to arthroplasty. Thus, if we re-create the patellar-trochlear relationship that we started with, appropriate patellar tracking will result; altering that relationship causes patellar maltracking.

Figure 13-1. The thickness of the anterior flange of the femoral component is 10 mm while the bone resected from the anterior femur is only 5 mm in thickness. This can lead to overstuffing of the patellofemoral joint.

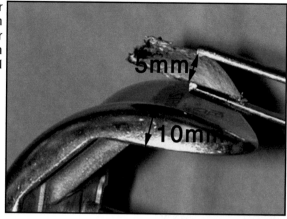

Figure 13-2. The anterior trochlear of a typical male patient is on the right and a female on the left. Notice the difference in the thickness of the anterior trochlear; the female is much thinner than the male. Subsequently, the anterior trochlear on some total knee systems have a women's option that will not overstuff the patellofemoral joint and better tracking will result as shown.

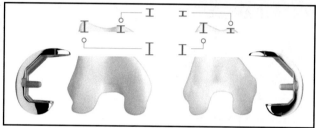

Problem: Overstuffing the Patellofemoral Joint

In general, the patella should be restored millimeter for millimeter with polyethylene. Overstuffing the patellofemoral joint will result in maltracking. A less commonly recognized problem, however, is that the patellofemoral joint can also be overstuffed by replacing more anterior femur than is resected. This is a particular problem in women, where the anterior trochlea is oftentimes not as thick as the standard component that replaces it (Figure 13-1). Therefore, for many women, the anterior trochlear is overstuffed unless a specially designed (women's) knee is used (Figure 13-2).

Problem: Femoral Component Rotation

Historically, the largest contributor to patellofemoral problems has been internal rotation of the femoral component.[1,2] However, in most modern systems, the instruments direct the surgeon to implant the femoral component with 3 degrees of external rotation relative to the posterior condyles. However, a more accurate method of rotating the femoral component is to align it parallel to the epicondylar axis; a line from the prominence of the lateral epicondyle to the sulcus of the medial epicondyle.[3]

The epicondylar axis is particularly helpful in the valgus knee since referencing the deficient posterior lateral condyles will result in an internally rotated femoral component. Additionally, a useful intraoperative sign to ensure that appropriate femoral cuts

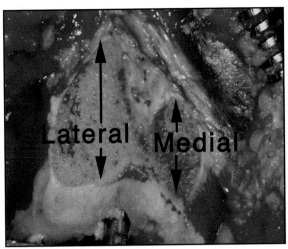

Figure 13-3. View of the cut anterior surface of the distal femur (right knee). The exposed bone on the lateral side is substantially longer in length as compared to the medial side, indicating appropriate external rotation of the femoral cuts.

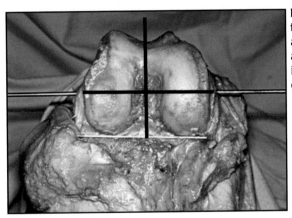

Figure 13-4. Whitesides line is drawn in the deepest part of the trochlear recess and is perpendicular to the epicondylar axis, which has been marked with pins in the center of the medial and lateral epicondyles.

have been made is the anterior trochlear groove; more bone should be removed from the lateral than the medial anterior trochlear (Figure 13-3). If the exposed bone on the medial side is equal in length to the lateral side, then the femoral component is internally rotated. Lastly, Whiteside's Line, which is the deepest part of the trochlear recess, should be perpendicular to the epicondylar axis and is a useful final check to ensure that the femoral component is oriented appropriately (Figure 13-4).

Problem: Femoral Component Placement

A femoral component that is placed medially will translate the trochlear groove medial and result in lateral patellar tracking. Therefore, the femur should be placed as close to the lateral edge of the exposed bone as possible. However, it is important not to allow the component to overhang laterally, tenting the lateral retinaculum and resulting in pain and poor patella tracking. This is a particular problem in many women where the anterior trochlea is not as wide as the standard component that replaces it (Figure 13-5A). Some total knee systems have a women's option that will not overhang the trochlear and will obviate these problems (Figure 13-5A). In addition, these female-specific components also

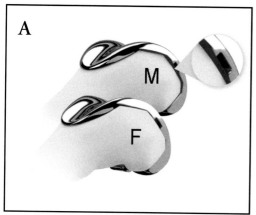 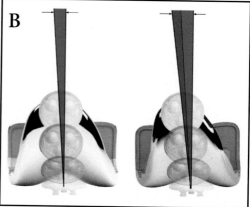

Figure 13-5. (A) Lateral view of a female femur. In many women the trochlea is not as wide as the standard (male M) component and symptomatic overhang occurs. Specially designed (female) components will for many women result in no overhang and obviate these problems. (B) The trochlea angle of a standard and female-specific component. The female-specific component have a trochlear angle that is larger to help guide the patella in women, more closely matching the female "Q-angle," which is larger than the male Q-angle.

have a trochlear angle that is larger to help guide the patella in women, more closely matching the female "Q-angle," which is larger than the male Q-angle (Figure 13-5B).

Problem: The Tibial Component

The proper rotational orientation of the tibial component is to be aligned with the center of the medial one-third of the tibial tubercle.[2] Intraoperatively, a pin can be placed at the tibial tubercle and aimed toward the PCL. Then, the component is placed 18 degrees internal to the tip of the tibial tubercle (this is 3 minutes on a clock face).[1] This point then corresponds roughly with the center of the medial 1/3; however, it is a much more reproducible mark (Figure 13-6). A secondary check is to notice that when the tibia is properly rotated, it is flush posterolateral on the tibial plateau and there will be some posteromedial bone, which is uncovered. Lastly, lateral placement of the tibial component also improves patellofemoral tracking.

Problem: The Patellar Component

Placing the patella button medially on the native patella helps patellofemoral tracking. Furthermore, any remaining bone on the lateral side of the native patella should be removed to avoid tenting the retinaculum and later impingement and pain from this bone.

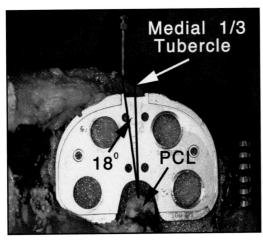

Figure 13-6. Guidelines for obtaining appropriate external rotation of the tibial component. A pin is placed in the tibial tubercle at the tip and aimed toward the PCL. This determines the orientation of the tibia. The component is then placed 18 degrees internal to the tip of the tibial tubercle (3 minutes on a clock face). This point corresponds roughly with the center of the medial 1/3 of the tibial tubercle. When the tibial component has been appropriately externally rotated, the posteromedial portion of the proximal tibia is uncovered.

Trialing

After all of the components are in place, a trial reduction should be performed to assess patellofemoral tracking. This assessment should be done without towel clips holding the arthrotomy together. If there is any concern about patellofemoral tracking, the surgeon must determine which component or components have been malpositioned or malrotated.

References

1. Berger RA, Crossett LS, Jacobs JJ, Rubash HE. Malrotation causing patellofemoral complications after total knee arthroplasty. *Clin Orthop.* 1998;(356):144.
2. Insall JN, Binazzi R, Soudry M, Mestriner LA. Total knee arthroplasty. *Clin Orthop.* 1985;(192):13.
3. Berger RA, Rubash HE, Seel MJ, Thompson WH, Crossett LS. Determining the rotational alignment of the femoral component in total knee arthroplasty using the epicondylar axis. *Clin Orthop.* 1993;(286):40.

How Do You Determine Appropriate Femoral Component Rotation at the Time of Surgery?

Richard Illgen II, MD
Matthew Squire, MD, MS

Femoral component rotation in total knee replacement is important to optimize patello-femoral and tibiofemoral kinematics.[1,2] Several reference axes exist to establish femoral rotation, but debate continues with regard to which axis most accurately and reproducibly establishes optimal rotational alignment.[3] The three most commonly used reference axes include the posterior femoral condylar axis, the transepicondylar axis, and the anterior-posterior axis (AP axis, Whiteside's Line) (Figure 14-1).[4] The AP axis is defined as a line that extends through the central axis of the femoral trochlear groove ending centrally in the femoral condylar notch. The epicondylar axis is a line connecting the midpoint of the medial and lateral femoral epicondyles. The lateral epicondyle is a discrete structure that can generally be palpated without difficulty, but the medial epicondyle has two peaks and a sulcus. The epicondylar axis runs between the mid-point of the lateral epicondyle and the midpoint of the medial epicondyle as defined by the medial epicondylar sulcus (see Figure 14-1).[1-3] The posterior condylar axis is a line defined by the posterior aspect of the medial and lateral femoral condyles (see Figure 14-1).

It is important to recognize the normal relationship between the AP, epicondylar, and posterior condylar axes. The AP axis is generally perpendicular to the epicondylar axis and the posterior condylar axis is internally rotated 3 degrees relative to the epicondylar axis (see Figure 14-1). However, significant individual variability exists with regard to the amount of femoral rotation relative to the posterior condylar axis, particularly comparing male and female femurs. Debate also continues regarding the reproducibility of the epicondylar axis as a reference and its use in minimally invasive total knee arthoplasty (TKA) is limited due to the reduced surgical exposure. The more complex the case, the more important it is for the surgeon to utilize a redundant system and multiple intraoperative landmarks to establish appropriate femoral rotation. It is therefore important for treating clinicians to understand the limitations of each axis and make appropriate intraoperative adjustments to ensure that anatomic rotation is restored.

Figure 14-1. Intraoperative photograph during total knee arthroplasty demonstrating the epicondylar axis, the anterior-posterior axis, and posterior condylar axis of the knee.

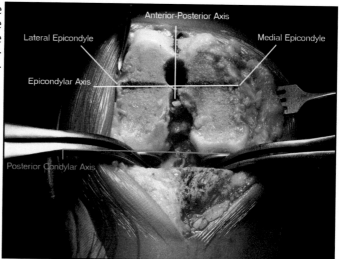

Figure 14-2. Intraoperative photograph during total knee arthroplasty demonstrating the femoral rotation established with the balanced tension technique. The femoral component is placed parallel with the cut tibial surface with the collateral ligaments placed under tension using laminar spreaders.

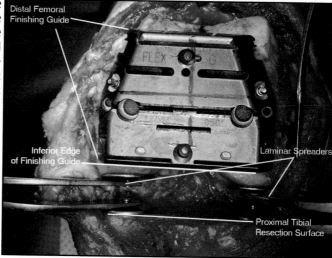

In some cases, the posterior condyles do not represent a reliable reference for rotation due to arthritic deformity in primary TKA or bone loss in revision TKA. In primary TKA, the most common challenge for establishing appropriate femoral rotation occurs in the valgus knee with a hypoplastic lateral femoral condyle. In these cases, using the posterior femoral condyles alone to establish femoral rotation can often lead to internal rotation of the femoral component and therefore patellar maltracking. In these cases, it is important to use another reference axis such as the AP axis and/or the epicondylar axis to establish appropriate femoral rotation.[4] In revision TKA, there is often asymmetric bone loss of the posterior femoral condyles and destruction of the normal landmarks that establish the AP axis. In these cases, it is often appropriate to use the epicondylar axis to establish femoral rotation.

An alternative method to establish appropriate femoral rotation involves using a ligament tensioning device (Figure 14-2). In this method, the tibial cut is made first perpendicular to the mechanical axis of the knee. All ligament balancing is then completed with the knee in extension to establish a symmetric rectangular extension gap. The knee is then flexed and devices such as laminar spreaders are utilized to apply symmetric tension to the medial and lateral aspects of the knee in flexion (see Figure 14-2). The femoral finishing guide is then applied to the distal femur with the tension devices in place to establish an appropriate rectangular flexion gap that is symmetric with the gap established in extension.[5] This technique can be used in both primary and revision TKA and has been shown to be an effective and accurate method of establishing femoral rotation.[5]

Controversy continues regarding the most reliable method to achieve femoral component rotation. In experienced hands, femoral component rotation can reliably be achieved using the aforementioned techniques in the majority of cases. However, even in experienced hands using proven techniques outliers remain that demonstrate femoral component rotation in suboptimal position. No method appears to be clearly superior to avoid outliers in femoral rotation. Navigation techniques have been shown to improve axial and sagittal alignment in primary TKA.[6] However, to date, navigation has been less successful in improving the accuracy of achieving appropriate femoral rotation. Further research is needed in this area.

References

1. Miller MC, Berger RA, Petrella AJ, et al. Optimizing femoral component rotation in total knee arthroplasty. *Clin Orthop Relat Res.* 2001;38-45.
2. Berger RA, Crossett LS, Jacobs JJ, et al. Malrotation causing patellofemoral complications after total knee arthroplasty. *Clin Orthop Relat Res.* 1998;144-153.
3. Berger RA, Rubash HE, Seel MJ, et al. Determining the rotational alignment of the femoral component in total knee arthroplasty using the epicondylar axis. *Clin Orthop Relat Res.* 1993;40-47.
4. Whiteside LA, Arima J. The anteroposterior axis for femoral rotational alignment in valgus total knee arthroplasty. *Clin Orthop Relat Res.* 1995;168-172.
5. Fehring TK. Rotational malalignment of the femoral component in total knee arthroplasty. *Clin Orthop Relat Res.* 2000;72-79.
6. Chin PL, Yang KY, Yeo SJ, et al. Randomized control trial comparing radiographic total knee arthroplasty implant placement using computer navigation versus conventional technique. *J Arthroplasty.* 2005;20:618-626.

HOW DO I DETERMINE TIBIAL COMPONENT ROTATION IN TOTAL KNEE ARTHROPLASTY?

David Manning, MD
Seann Carr, MD

There are two fundamental goals to consider when discussing the optimal placement of the tibial component during total knee arthoplasty (TKA). My first goal is to prevent component subsidence by transmitting weight bearing forces to the largest possible surface area of bone. I prefer part of the load to be applied to the cortical rim of the proximal osteotomized tibia.[1-3] Optimal load transfer is achieved through a combination of component sizing and rotation. My second goal is to affect tibial-femoral and patella-femoral kinematics through the influence of tibial component rotation on the reconstruction Q-angle.[3] The importance of tibial component rotation on the reconstruction Q angle is often overstated. Femoral rotation is far more influential on the overall kinematics of a total knee replacement. The deleterious effects created by an improperly, internally rotated femoral component cannot be corrected by any amount of tibial rotation.[2]

I note bearing surface geometry and design (round on flat vs semiconforming, and rotating vs fixed) when considering the effect of tibial implant rotation on tibial–femoral and patella–femoral kinematics. Round on flat, fixed bearing configurations, and rotating platform bearings allow for rotation through the joint. This minimizes the effect of tibial component rotation on the reconstruction Q angle. The opposite extreme is a fixed bearing, varus–valgus stabilizing implant in which little to no rotation occurs through the joint. In this case, improper tibial component rotation negatively impacts patella–femoral kinematics as well as distal extremity cosmesis. For the purpose of this discussion, I prefer to use a symmetric modular tibial baseplate with a fixed semi-conforming, posterior substituting bearing surface. I surgically address the more important femoral component rotation first. I rely predominantly on the accurate and repeatable landmarks of Whiteside's Line and the trans-epicondylar axis.[1] The properly positioned femur, and how it relates to the tibial bearing, may be used to evaluate tibial rotation.

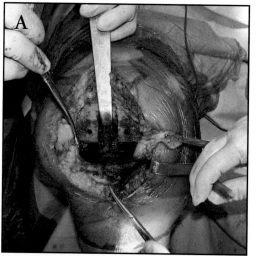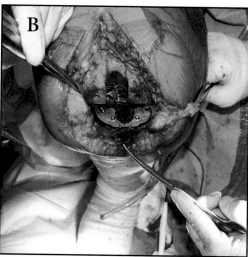

Figure 15-1. (A) Marking of proximal tibia to depict midcoronal axis and perpendicular line oriented toward middle-medial third junction of the tibial tubercle. (B) Midsagittal axis of properly rotated tibial component is parallel to the perpendicular line oriented toward the middle-medial third junction of the tibial tubercle. Note that the midsagital axis of the tibial trial is also oriented parallel to the tibial crest over the first ray of the foot. In each picture a hemostat marks the middle-medial third junction of the tibial tubercle.

There are multiple checks I do to ensure the tibial base plate is appropriately aligned. I evaluate the component based on both anatomic and prosthetic factors. After choosing an appropriately sized implant, my preferred anatomic check is to align the tibial base plate with the junction of the medial and middle thirds of the tibial tubercle[1,3] (Figure 15-1). This alignment should be done through rotation and not simple translation in the coronal plane. This rotation should create minimal posterior-medial tibial plateau uncovering. Additionally, this maneuver achieves optimal anterior medial and posterior lateral cortical contact thereby optimizing load transfer and minimizing the risk of subsidence. Simple translation of the trial implant results in undersizing, medial, or lateral tibial uncovering and suboptimal load transfer to bone. An alternative anatomic method is to mark the osteotomized tibial surface along its coronal axis. I then draw a perpendicular line in the direction of the medial-middle third junction of the tibial tubercle. This perpendicular is usually parallel with the midsagittal axis of a properly rotated symmetric tibial baseplate[3] (see Figure 15-1). My final anatomic check includes an extramedullary alignment rod outrigged from the pinned tibial base plate. The rod should overlay the medial-middle third junction of the tibial tubercle, the center of the ankle mortise, as well as point to the first ray of a neutrally aligned foot[3] (see Figure 15-1).

I then proceed to evaluate my prosthetic cues for assessing tibial rotation. These are based on the relationship between the properly placed femoral component and the semi-congruent or dished bearing surface. I perform my trial reduction with the tibial tray pinned in rotation dictated by my interpretation of the anatomy as described earlier. With the knee reduced and in full extension there should be absolute congruence of the femoral component and the anterior edge of the semi-congruent bearing surface (Figure 15-2). Edge loading should not be tolerated. I then flex the knee and observe both the femoral–tibial bearing interaction as well as patellar tracking. At 90 degrees of flexion with modest

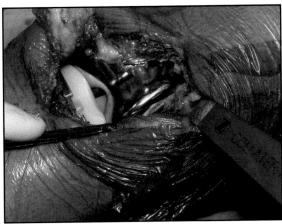

Figure 15-2. Rotational congruence is seen between the femoral component and the anterior edge or this semicongruous polyethylene bearing surface. Improper rotation of the tibial component would result in edge loading of the polyethylene. I find this check of rotation very helpful during minimally invasive TKA as the anatomy is not clearly visible during all stages of the procedure.

load applied to the joint, the bearing should again be congruent and without edge loading. "Hands free" patellar tracking should be free from tilt, subluxation, or dislocation.

If I observe congruence but patellar tracking is suboptimal, simply reorienting the tibia will not achieve the desired improvement. I correct patellar tracking by examining and repositioning the femur if necessary, assessing patellar component placement, and/or performing soft tissue release laterally. I address good "hands free" patellar tracking with suboptimal femoral-tibial congruence by unpinning the tibial trial and cycling the knee. With this technique the femoral component coupled with a dished polyethylene bearing surface can dictate an improved tibial rotation.

I find these multiple checks to set tibial component rotation during TKA to be successful, repeatable, rapid, and simple.

References

1. Uehara K, Kadoya Y, Kobayashi A, Ohashi H, Yamano Y. Bone anatomy and rotational alignment in total knee arthroplasty. *CORR.* 2002 Sep;402:196-201.
2. Eckhoff DG, Metzger RG, Vandewalle MV. Malrotation associated with implant alignment technique in total knee arthroplasty. *CORR.* 1995 Dec;321:28-31.
3. Insall JN. Technique of total knee replacement. *AAOS Instr Course Lect.* 1981;30:324.

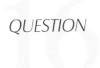
How Do I Perform a Lateral Release?

Mark D. Campbell, MD

Before I discuss how I do a lateral release it is important to discuss the indications for the procedure. A lateral release should be a tool at your disposal but should not be done without a clear understanding of why it is needed. It is also important to understand potential risks and complications associated with a lateral release. I personally have a very low lateral release rate, and as shown in a majority of the literature they are not routinely needed.[1]

As discussed in previous questions, component positioning has critical implications on patellofemoral tracking. Proper femoral and tibial rotation, as well as medialization of the patellar component will aid in proper tracking and is critical in clinical success. These basic principles must be observed before adjusting the extensor mechanism to improve tracking. A lateral release should not be used to make up for mistakes earlier in the operation.

Patellar Blood Supply

As apposed to lateral release done in native knees, lateral release in total knee arthroplasty is usually done in conjunction with a medial based arthrotomy, placing the patellar blood supply at even greater risk.[2] The major blood supply to the patella is represented by a vascular anastomotic ring (patellar plexus) lying just anterior to the rectus fibers and lying over the anterior patella. This ring is supplied by the genicular arteries (supreme, lateral superior and medial superior, lateral inferior, and medial inferior). Damage to the mid patellar vessels may predispose to patella ischemia. The anterior and posterior tibial recurrent arteries also add to the supply.

Figure 16-1. Single stitch technique. Note patella-femoral articulation is easily visualized.

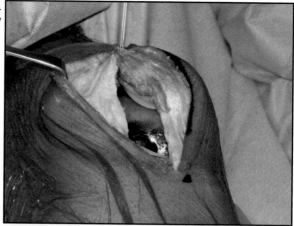

Figure 16-2. Excessive use of external pressure can falsely give the appearance of adequate tracking.

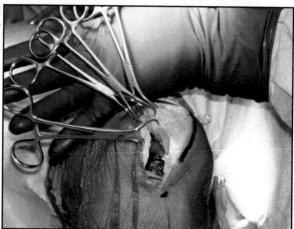

Preoperative Planning

A merchant view that shows good tracking preoperatively added to good component positioning during the procedure should rarely result in the need for lateral release. Good tracking on preoperative merchant views and a need for lateral release likely represents component malpositioning during the case. Lateral tracking on preoperative views should alert the physician to possible need for a lateral release. In virtually all studies the need for a lateral release is higher with a preoperative valgus deformity.[3]

Intraoperative Evaluation

Once all components have been placed (either trials or real components) patellar tracking can be assessed. I prefer to use a single retinacular closing stitch at the superior medial arthrotomy (Figure 16-1). With this technique I am not falsely correcting tracking problems and at the same time can visualize the patellofemoral dynamics directly. It is at this time that I can decide if a lateral release will improve my patellofemoral tracking. I believe that tracking should be assessed with minimal external pressure being applied

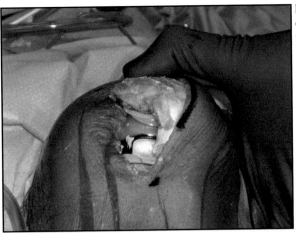

Figure 16-3. With manual correction, it can be difficult to regulate the amount of pressure being applied.

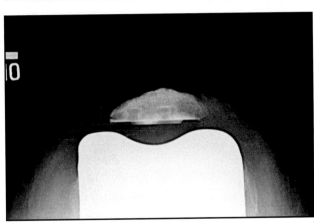

Figure 16-4. Note lateral facet removed and balanced patella-femoral tracking.

(such as excessive manual pressure, towel clips, or multiple sutures) (Figures 16-2 and 16-3). Although popular, the "no touch" technique will result in over utilization of a lateral release if every patella that tilts or subluxes is treated.[1]

How to Do a Lateral Release

My preferred technique is an "outside in" release. At the time of resurfacing, I remove bone from the lateral facet, until flush with the patellar button. In addition to removing bone that may impinge, I am "untethering" the lateral retinaculum at the same time, functionally lengthening the lateral retinaculum. (Figure 16-4)

If a formal release is required I release the retinaculum at least one centimeter lateral to patella and every attempt is made to start the release distal to the superior lateral retinacular artery, thus preserving this important blood supply. I use electro-cautery in performing this release and my testing of patella-femoral tracking after is the same as previously described.

It has been shown that tourniquet use can affect patellar tracking. Studies suggest that deflation of the tourniquet before lateral release can improve tracking and obviate the

Figure 16-5. Multiple stab incisions allow the lateral retinalculum to be effectively "lengthened."

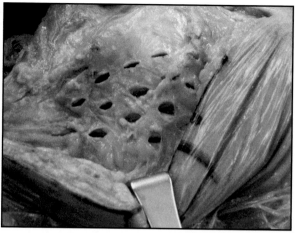

need for release.[4,5] I release the tourniquet if I am contemplating the need for a release and often find the release not needed.

Inside Out

The inside out technique is similar to the aforementioned, however the inner retinaculum must be visualized and usually requires patellar eversion. This may be more difficult in some less invasive exposures but allows direct visualization, and easier protection of the components.

Pie Crusting/Meshing

The pie-crusting technique achieves the goals of the lateral release with a theoretical reduction in postoperative morbidity. This technique consists of multiple, longitudinal, parallel 5 to 10 mm stab incisions to mesh and expand the lateral retinaculum, thereby medializing the patella[6] (Figure 16-5).

Complications Associated with a Lateral Release

In most studies, complications associated with lateral release are rare.[7] When occurring, most are thought to be related to interruption of patellar blood supply. The most common complications associated with lateral release are patellar fractures and patellar component loosening.[8]

References

1. Benjamin J, Chelvers M. Correcting lateral patellar tilt at the time of total knee arthroplasty can result in over-use of lateral release. *Arthroplasty.* 2006 Sep;21(6)(Suppl 2):121-126.
2. Scuderi G, Scharf SC, Meltzer LP, Scott WN. The relationship of lateral releases to patella viability in total knee arthroplasty. *J Arthroplasty.* 1987;2(3):209-214.
3. Laskin RS. Lateral release rates after total knee arthroplasty. Clin Orthop Res. 2001;(392):88-93.

4. Lombari AV Jr, Berend KR, Mallory TH, Dodds KL, Adams JB. The relationship of lateral release and tourniquet deflation in total knee arthroplasty. *J Knee Surg*. 2003;16(4):209-214.
5. Marson BM, Tokish JT. The effect of a tourniquet on intraoperative patellofemoral tracking during total knee arthroplasty. *Arthroplasty*. 1999;14(2):197-199.
6. Healy WL, Iorio R, Warren P. Mesh expansion release of the lateral patellar retinaculum during total knee arthroplasty. *J Bone Joint Surg Am*. 2004;86A(Suppl 1, Pt 2):193-200.
7. Weber AB, Worland RL, Jessup DE, Van Bowen J, Keenan J. The consequences of lateral release in total knee replacement: a review of over 1000 knees with follow up between 5 and 11 years. *Knee*. 2003;10(2):187-191.
8. Ritter MA, Pierce MJ, Zhou H, Meding JB, Faris PM. Patellar complication (total knee arthroplasty). Effect of lateral release and thickness. *Clin Orthop Relat Res*. 1999;(367):149-157.

THE FEMORAL COMPONENT SIZING GUIDE IS MEASURING BETWEEN TWO SIZES. SHOULD I CHOOSE THE SMALLER OR LARGER SIZE?

Frank R. DiMaio, MD

Before answering the proposed question, it is imperative that you understand the consequences of improperly sizing the femoral component at the time of total knee arthroplasty.

In general, choosing a femoral component too large for the patient's femoral anatomy (oversizing) may lead to postoperative stiffness. Oversizing the femur in the antero-posterior (AP) dimension results in "overstuffing" the patello-femoral joint and increases the distance that the extensor mechanism and patella needs to travel during flexion. Poor postoperative flexion is the consequence. Over-sizing the femoral component in the mediolateral (ML) dimension may also contribute to postoperative stiffness, as well as collateral soft tissue impingement and pain relating to component overhang.

On the contrary, choosing a femoral component too small for the patient's anatomy (under-sizing) may lead to flexion instability. Recreating the AP dimension is paramount for soft tissue and collateral tension and flexion gap balance. Moreover, under-sizing is one of the most common reasons for anterior femoral notching, particularly if excessive external rotation is applied during femoral preparation.

The decision whether I choose the size larger or smaller than the femoral sizing guide indicates, depends on which referencing guide I utilize at this step.

Many manufacturers include both posterior and anterior referencing distal femoral sizing guides in their instrument sets. I prefer to use a posterior referencing guide for the majority of my cases. With this type guide, the "feet" of the guide are placed under the exposed posterior femoral condyles with the knee in adequate flexion (Figure 17-1). Next, a stylus is dropped onto the anterior cortex of the distal femur and the AP dimension

Figure 17-1. An example of a posterior referencing femoral sizing guide applied to the prepared distal femur.

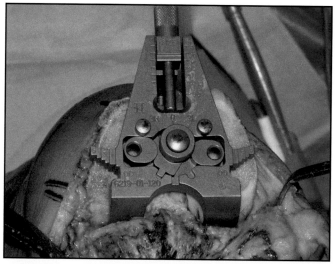

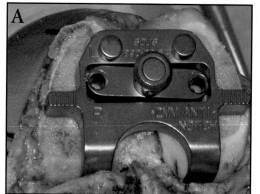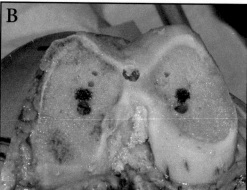

Figure 17-2. (A) Application of a 2-mm anti-notch guide. (B) The marker ink depicts 2 mm of translation of the fixation drill holes to prevent notching f the anterior femoral cortex upon final preparation.

determined. This method is reliable to restore the joint line in flexion, balance the PCL in cruciate-retaining cases, and minimize the risk of flexion instability. When between sizes with a posterior referencing guide, I typically choose the larger size, so as to avoid anterior distal femoral notching. If I believe that the anterior phalange of the larger size component will be too proud, or if the ML diameter is too wide, then I consider one of two options.

My first choice is to translate the distal femoral condylar cutting block 2 mm anteriorly. This translation usually allows me to accommodate the femur to the smaller size and avoids a "close call" if notching is suspected otherwise. This variation in technique can be performed with an "anti-notch" guide (Figure 17-2) and will theoretically increase the flexion gap by 2 mm; this is usually well tolerated in most cases with little, if any, kinematic consequence.

My second choice is to re-prepare the distal femur in 3 degrees of flexion to allow for a smaller size component without notching. This variation is easily achieved with a semi-custom distal femoral cutting block, which is readily available by many of the manufacturers (Figure 17-3). Slight flexion of the femoral component is well tolerated and rarely results

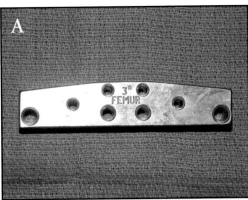 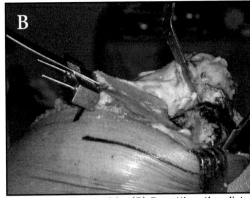

Figure 17-3. (A) A sample of a custom 3 degree femoral cutting guide. (B) Recutting the distal femur in 3 degrees of flexion in order to prevent notching of the anterior distal femoral cortex.

in loss of knee extension if no more than 3 degrees is built into the distal resection. I would not recommend this alteration if the patient has a pre-operative flexion contracture.

In the rare cases in which I employ an anterior referencing sizing guide, I typically choose the smaller of the options when the guide measures between sizes. The potential risk here is not notching, but rather resecting too much posterior condyle. These guides rest a stylus onto the anterior distal femoral cortex and measure down along the posterior condyles. Resection of excessive posterior femoral condyle theoretically results in a larger flexion gap, and potential flexion instability. This scenario is usually encountered when an anterior referencing guide is employed in a severe varus knee with a hypertrophic, distorted medial femoral condyle. In this scenario, more than an anatomic amount of posterior condyle may be resected medially, and may make flexion gap balancing a challenge.

References

1. Guyton JL, Rosenberg AG. The Miller-Galante total knee arthroplasty: Evolution of design, surgical technique, and clinical results. *Techniques in Orthopaedics*. 1991 Dec;6(4):30-38.
2. Scott RD. Primary total knee arthroplasty surgical technique. Chapter 4. *Total Knee Arthroplasty*. Saunders, Philadelphia, PA; 2006:20-38.

WHAT IS FLEXION INSTABILITY AND HOW DO I PREVENT IT DURING TOTAL KNEE ARTHROPLASTY?

David J. Jacofsky, MD

Presentation

Patients with postoperative flexion instability most commonly complain of pain in the region of the pes anserine bursa, as well as the distal iliotibial band. This may initially be diagnosed as "idiopathic" bursitis, although in reality the etiology is flexion instability. The patients typically report increased pain and weakness with stair climbing and may report recurrent knee effusion

To diagnose this postoperatively, I sit the patient in a chair, flex the knee to 90 degrees, place the patient's foot between mine, and shuck the tibia anteriorly and posteriorly (Figure 18-1). Some excursion occurs in all patients, but if this excursion is greater than 5 to 10 mm *and* clinically reproduces the patient's symptoms, then flexion instability is present.

If the symptoms began immediately after surgery, it is likely due to a technical error as discussed later. If, however, it occurs late, it may be due to attrition or rupture of a previously competent posterior cruciate ligament in a cruciating retaining knee arthroplasty.

Etiology (Table 18-1)

Flexion instability occurs when the flexion gap is larger than the extension gap. This may be due to a number of factors. A relatively tight extension gap may occur due to under-resection of the distal femur, mandating a relatively thin polyethylene insert to achieve full extension, thus causing flexion instability due to a relatively loose gap in

Table 18-1

Causes of Flexion Instability

Femoral Side

Tight extension gap (under-resection distal femur)
Extension of femoral component
Undersizing of femoral component (over-resection of posterior condyles)
Anteriorization of femoral component (over-resection of posterior condyles)

Tibial Side

Excessive tibial slope
Relatively flat tibial insert geometry

PCL

Attrition or incompetence
Delayed rupture
Over-recession

Figure 18-1. Physical exam technique to test for flexion instability.

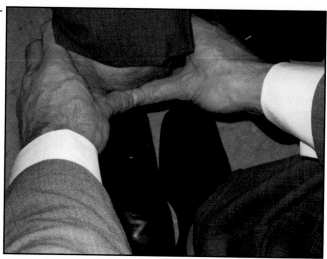

flexion. Conversely, an appropriate extension gap can exist, but over-resection of the posterior femur and/or undersizing or anteriorizing of the femoral component will also lead to a relatively large flexion gap. This most easily occurs inadvertently when one uses an anterior referencing system to size the femoral component, especially if when between sizes the smaller size is chosen. This can lead to resection of more posterior bone than is replaced with the implant. It is for this reason that many prefer a posterior referencing system, thus maintaining a constant resection of posterior condylar bone.

Excessive tibial slope can also exacerbate instability in flexion. Although flexion instability is more common with the use of a cruciate retaining implant, a poorly balanced flexion gap will lead to symptomatic flexion instability even in a posterior sta-

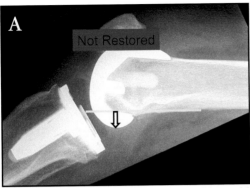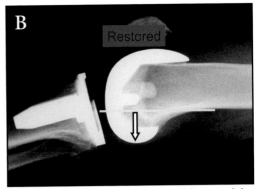

Figure 18-2. (A) Lateral radiograph of a total knee arthroplasty in which the posterior condylar offset has not been restored. This patient suffered from flexion instability. (B) Lateral radiograph of a total knee arthroplasty in which the posterior condylar offset has been restored.

bilized knee replacement. In my referral revision practice, flexion instability has now become the most common etiology for symptomatic failure of total knee replacement requiring revision.

Management

Initially an attempt can be made to treat patients nonoperatively with corticosteroid injections into the pes tendons or casting in extension for 4 to 6 weeks. In my experience, over half of patients initially managed successfully nonoperatively eventually develop recurrence.

If revision is indicated, conversion of a cruciate retaining implant to a cruciate substituting design is usually successful. Flexion instability in a cruciate substituting implant requires either femoral revision to adequately balance the gaps, or if global instability is present, conversion to a rotating hinge prosthesis.

Intraoperatively, it is imperative that one checks for stability in flexion. In general, due to the large forces across the knee with weight bearing activities, the gap will appear looser after surgery than it does intraoperatively. This is counterintuitive, as one often thinks that closure of the knee will improve the knee's stability in flexion. However, one should never rely on the extensor mechanism closure to provide stability in this regard.

If flexion instability is present recheck all osseous cuts. Confirm that the distal femur was not under-resected, and recheck implant sizing. One may need to either posteriorize or upsize the femoral component to balance the gaps. Preoperative radiographs can be helpful in making certain that the posterior offset of the knee is restored (Figures 18-2A, 18-2B). Additionally, the resected posterior bone can be measured with a caliper to confirm that they are thinner or equal to the posterior thickness of the implant to be used. Upsizing at this point may require the use of posterior wedges or additional cement fill about the posterior aspect of the condyles.

If the bony cuts and implant sizing seem appropriate, then one needs to evaluate the soft tissues. If a CR knee is being used, conversion to a PS implant will

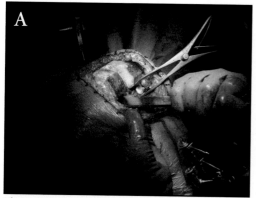 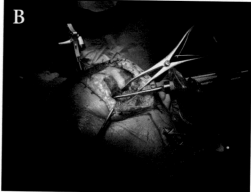

Figure 18-3. Intraoperative images of the use of a laminar speader and an psteotome to carefully strip the posterior capsule from the posterior aspect of the femur to increase the size of the extension gap.

Figure 18-4. Intraoperative computer navigation data showing the size of the extension gap when the knee is fully extended.

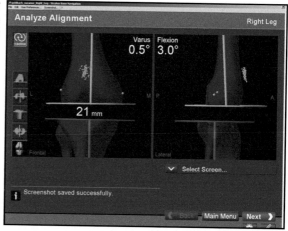

improve stability in flexion if the PCL is attenuated or has been over-released. If the imbalance is not too great, stripping the posterior capsule from the femur will often enlarge the extension gap allowing a thicker polyethylene insert to be placed and improve stability in flexion (Figure 18-3). If this alone does not work, then either slight elevation of the joint line (especially in patients with a preoperative flexion contracture of more than 10 degrees) or upsizing of the femoral component is required.

In my practice, the use of computer navigation has assisted me to ensure appropriate osseous resection and confirm the presence of a balanced knee. Navigation software will now inform the surgeon of the exact size of the flexion gap and the extension gaps. I prefer a flexion gap that is 1 to 2 mm smaller than the extension gap in the nonweight bearing assessment of the trials in surgery (Figures 18-4 and 18-5). Other devices, such as tensiometers and spacer blocks, are also available. Whatever the method and implant a surgeon prefers, imbalance of the gaps at the time of surgical closure will most often lead to an unsuccessful outcome.

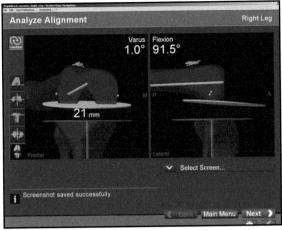

Figure 18-5. Intraoperative computer navigation data showing the size of the flexion gap when the knee is flexed 90 degrees. Note the gap is equal to the extension gap (see Figure 18-4).

References

1. Romero J, Stahelin T, Binkert C, Pfirrmann C, Hodler J, Kessler O. The clinical consequences of flexion gap asymmetry in total knee arthroplasty. *J Arthroplasty*. 2007 Feb;22(2):235-240.
2. Mihalko WM, Krackow KA. Flexion and extension gap balancing in revision total knee arthroplasty. *Clin Orthop Relat Res*. 2006 May;446:121-126.
3. Schwab JH, Haidukewych GJ, Hanssen AD, Jacofsky DJ, Pagnano MW. Flexion instability without dislocation after posterior stabilized total knees. *Clin Orthop Relat Res*. 2005 Nov;440:96-100.
4. Whiteside LA. Ligament balancing in revision total knee arthroplasty. *Clin Orthop Relat Res*. 2004 Jun;(423):178-185.
5. McAuley JP, Engh GA, Ammeen DJ. Treatment of the unstable total knee arthroplasty. *Instr Course Lect*. 2004;53:237-241.
6. Nabeyama R, Matsuda S, Miura H, Kawano T, Nagamine R, Mawatari T, Tanaka K, Iwamoto Y. Changes in anteroposterior stability following total knee arthroplasty. *J Orthop Sci*. 2003;8(4):526-531.
7. Clarke HD, Scuderi GR. Flexion instability in primary total knee replacement. *J Knee Surg*. 2003 Apr;16(2):123-128.
8. Matsuda S, Miura H, Nagamine R, Urabe K, Matsunobu T, Iwamoto Y. Knee stability in posterior cruciate ligament retaining total knee arthroplasty. *Clin Orthop Relat Res*. 1999 Sep;(366):169-173.

I AM DOING A TOTAL KNEE IN A PATIENT WITH A VARUS DEFORMITY. I HAVE DONE MY STANDARD RELEASE AND THE KNEE IS STILL TIGHT MEDIALLY. WHAT SHOULD I DO?

Gregg R. Klein, MD
Mark A. Hartzband, MD

Varus deformity accounts for approximately 85% of arthritic knee patterns. It is created by progressive loss of the medial articular cartilage and bone followed by progressive contracture of the medial soft tissues and, ultimately, attenuation of the lateral soft tissues. When preoperative standing films show lateral subluxation of the tibia on the femur, one should anticipate the need for more extensive releases and the possible need for a constrained implant. In addition, flexion contracture is often associated with varus deformity and must be dealt with concomitantly as an integrated part of the medial release.

The tension stress evaluation forms the basis for ligament balancing in total knee arthoplasty (TKA). It refers to the process whereby the contracted soft tissues are released until they are symmetric with the contralateral soft tissues. This process converts an initially trapezoid flexion or extension gap into a rectangular gap. The goal is rectangular flexion and extension gaps that are within 1 to 2 mm of each other.

Regardless of the order, it is imperative that the release is sequential. The symmetry or asymmetry of the gap must be repeatedly assessed as the release proceeds in order to prevent over-release of the contracted soft tissues.

Figure 19-1. Release of the proximal superficial MCL.

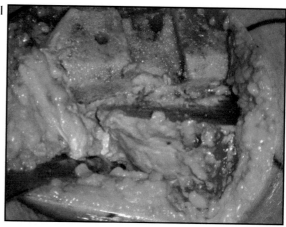

Technique

We first perform a standard arthrotomy with anteromedial release. A sleeve of soft tissue is released: including the deep media collateral ligament (MCL) and posteromedial capsule starting from the medial border of the patellar tendon and extending posteromedially. The distal extent of this release is approximately 8 mm below the joint line (or just distal to the tibial osteophytes). This exposure is usually carried to the posteromedial corner. Next, we remove the marginal medial tibial and femoral osteophytes that are accessible. Removing the osteophytes that are tenting the MCL relaxes the ligament and aids in balancing the gaps. The intimate relationship of the MCL to the medial joint line accounts for the significant medial soft tissue relaxation that occurs with simple osteophyte resection. This release of the deep MCL, posteromedial capsule and medial tibial and femoral osteophytes will balance approximately 85% of varus knees.

If further release is needed we slowly release the proximal portion of the superficial MCL (SMCL) approximately 2 to 3 cm below the joint line (Figure 19-1). The semimembranosus tendon, which is an active stabilizer of the medial knee, may be released next. The semimembranosus is released by externally rotating the tibia to identify the semimembranosus tendon, which inserts at the posteromedial corner of the tibia. Release of the semimembranosus tendon will aid in release of a flexion contracture as well as a varus contracture.

If additional medial release is required to obtain a balanced flexion and extension gap the medial proximal tibial metaphysis that extends beyond the medial border of the tibial tray may be trimmed in order take tension off the MCL. In fact, if more medial release is needed we may downsize the tibial component and lateralize it to the lateral tibial cortical margin (Figure 19-2). Downsizing the component will expose an additional 2 to 4 mm of medial metaphyseal bone (depending on the implant that is used), which can be resected from the medial proximal tibia.[1] It is easiest to remove the medial bone with a saw; however, the medial soft tissue structures must be protected. This downsizing and bone resection technique reduces the amount of soft tissue release necessary to balance the knee and thus minimizes the likelihood of over-release of the medial soft tissue that may occur with extensive distal SMCL and pes anserinus release. Theoretically, downsizing the component may result in greater forces across the knee. However, Dixon et al[1] have reported no adverse effects with this technique at an average follow-up of 42 months.

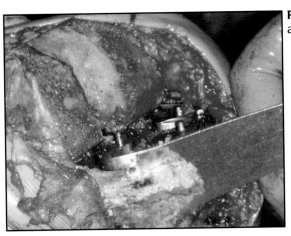

Figure 19-2. Medial tibial bone resection around the tibial trial.

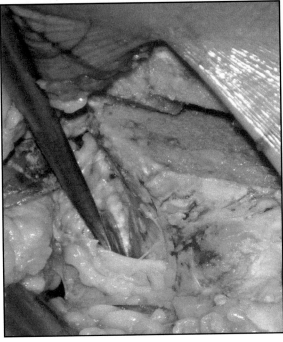

Figure 19-3. Release of the distal superficial MCL using a Cobb elevator.

The distal portion of the pes anserinus and the distal portion of the SMCL 8 to 10 cm below the joint line may be released (Figure 19-3) to obtain even greater medial soft tissue relaxation. This is best accomplished using a Cobb elevator or osteotome and running it down the tibial shaft thus raising a periosteal sleeve.

The SMCL is divided into two components: the vertically oriented anterior component and the obliquely oriented posterior component. The vertical component originates on the medial femoral condyle approximately 5 cm above the joint line and inserts posterior to the pes anserinus onto the proximal medial aspect of the tibia approximately 6 to 8 cm distal to the femoral tibial joint line. The two components of the SMCL serve different functions depending on the position of the knee. The anterior portion tightens in flexion whereas the posterior component loosens in flexion. Conversely, the anterior component is loose in extension whereas the posterior portion is tense in flexion.[2]

Figure 19-4. Soleal fibers of the superficial MCL.

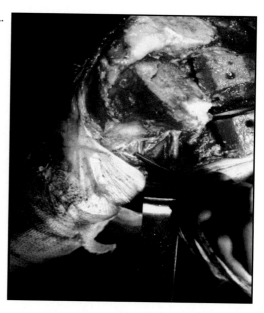

Remember to always stay anterior while releasing the SMCL to avoid completely detaching it. The pes anserinus may be released concomitantly with the SMCL sleeve if necessary. It is important to remember that release of the anterior portion of the SMCL preferentially creates laxity in flexion.[3] This differential laxity may be compounded by excessive external rotation of the femoral component due to the relative translation of the femoral insertion of the MCL posteriorly with femoral component external rotation. To avoid this complication of paradoxical posteromedial flexion instability, excessive external rotation of the femoral component in patients with severe varus deformity should be avoided.

In rare cases that are still not adequately balanced, release of the soleal fibers of the SMCL will create a major increase in medial soft tissue relaxation (Figure 19-4). The soleal fibers of the SMCL are the posteromedial fibers that blend imperceptibly with the soleal fascia. Often release of these fibers will create substantial laxity and a more constrained implant may be necessary.

Finally, if there is still medial soft tissue tightness a medial epicondylar osteotomy may be helpful.[4] However, this is only very rarely necessary. With the knee in 90 degrees of flexion, an osteotome may be use to osteotomize a wide based fragment. This elevates the collateral ligament origin and the adductor magnus tendon insertion. The osteotomized fragment can then be opened and translated posteriorly and distally. In addition, this technique provides improved exposure to the posterior aspect of the knee for further posterior capsular release for severe flexion contractures. After implantation of the components the fragment is distally translated as necessary for appropriate ligament tension (usually 1.5 to 2 cm). With the knee in 90 degrees of flexion, we fix the fragment in the translated position with 6.5 mm screw and washer.

Table 19-1
Sequence of Medial Soft Tissue Release

1. Deep MCL
2. Posteromedial capsule
3. Marginal medial tibial and femoral osteophytes
4. Superficial MCL—proximal portion
5. Semimembranosus
6. Medial Tibial bone resection
7. Superficial MCL—distal portion
8. Pes anserinus
9. Superficial MCL—soleal fibers
10. Medial epicondyle osteotomy

Conclusion

Although the majority of varus knee releases can be accomplished with a standard exposure a small percentage of primary knee arthroplasties will require additional soft tissue releases. Sequential release of the medial soft tissues as outlined (Table 19-1) will aid in obtaining a well-balanced knee with good long-term survival.

References

1. Dixon MC, Parsch D, Brown RR, Scott RD. The correction of severe varus deformity in total knee arthroplasty by tibial component downsizing and resection of uncapped proximal medial bone. *J Arthroplasty*. 2004;19:19-22.
2. Whiteside LA, Saeki K, Mihalko WM. Functional medical ligament balancing in total knee arthroplasty. *Clin Orthop Relat Res*. 2000:45-57.
3. Krackow KA, Mihalko WM. The effect of medial release on flexion and extension gaps in cadaveric knees: implications for soft-tissue balancing in total knee arthroplasty. *Am J Knee Surg*. 1999;12:222-8.
4. Engh GA, Ammeen D. Results of total knee arthroplasty with medial epicondylar osteotomy to correct varus deformity. *Clin Orthop Relat Res*. 1999:141-148.

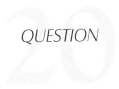
WHEN PERFORMING A TOTAL KNEE ARTHROPLASTY IN A PATIENT WITH A VALGUS DEFORMITY, WHAT STRUCTURES DO YOU RELEASE FIRST?

Keith R. Berend, MD

When attacking the valgus knee there are several principles that need to be addressed. The first is the approach. I routinely use a less-invasive, abbreviated median parapatellar approach, even with the valgus knee. I find the anatomy to be more familiar than with a lateral-based approach, and the less invasive instruments are designed to be applied from the medial side. Balancing the knee in flexion and extension and performing the necessary releases are relatively straightforward using this approach, and it is easily extensile into a more standard median parapatellar approach if needed.

It bears mentioning that the initial medial tibial exposure should be limited so as not to over release the medial side. Routinely, this means stopping the medial tibial exposure at or anterior to the superficial medial collateral ligament (MCL). Further exposure and/or medial release may be necessary, but can be performed in a graduated fashion during tibial preparation or balancing.

The next issue is the likelihood of combined deformities; namely valgus in association with a fixed flexion contracture. I would recommend cutting an additional 2 mm of distal femur if the knee has a significant (greater than 15 degrees) flexion contracture. Similarly, in the hyperflexible valgus knee with recurvatum, I would reduce the initial distal femoral resection by 2 mm.

I utilize a matched resection technique of total knee arthroplasty (TKA). In doing so, I perform the final balancing and soft tissue releases once the trial implants are placed. I routinely try to preserve the posterior cruciate ligament (PCL) as it can act as a secondary lateral stabilizer, especially in flexion. Preserving the PCL can allow for a more aggressive release of tight lateral structures when necessary.

Figure 20-1. The iliotibial band is released from anterior to posterior using electrocautery, just distal to the joint line, above Gerdy's tubercle. (Reproduced with permission of Joint Implant Surgeons, Inc.)

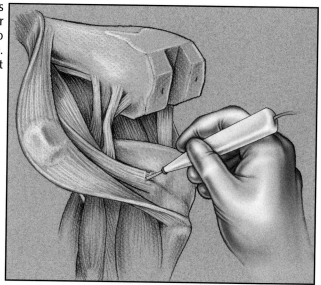

Once the trials are in place, the initial priority is to strive for full extension. It is necessary to clear osteophytes from the posterior recess of both the medial and lateral sides of the femur in order to obtain full extension and high flexion. If full extension is still not achieved, then the iliotibial (IT) band is released from anterior to posterior (Figure 20-1). This is performed just distal to the joint line, above Gerdy's tubercle. I would routinely use a tonsil clamp, dissecting between the subcutaneous tissue and the IT band. Electrocautery or a scalpel is then used to carefully release the entire structure. One size larger bearing may be required to balance the medial and lateral sides at this point.

Second, the knee is then flexed with only the tibial trial in place. A laminar spreader is used to distract the medial and lateral sides in flexion. If the flexion space is not rectangular and the lateral side is the tight side, then palpation of the tight lateral structures is done and the tightest structure released. This is usually the popliteus tendon (Figure 20-2). If the knee is still tight laterally, the laminar spreader is inserted in extension and the posterior capsule and lateral collateral ligament are lengthened through careful pie crusting (Figure 20-3). Highly constrained components should be available in case over-release results in lateral instability. This is another driving factor for why I prefer to use a cruciate retaining (CR) design, as cam and post instability can result if the lateral side is over-released.

Trials are inserted and stability and range of motion tested. If further releases are necessary, I then release the PCL. Again, this may require insertion of a thicker bearing with a cam and post or a more highly conforming, so-called deep dish polyethylene insert.

Be sure lateral flexion instability is not present; otherwise, a constrained bearing may need to be used. Finally, the medial-sided soft tissue sleeve may require further release at this point if the lateral side becomes more lax than the medial side. Avoid the "joint-jack" phenomenon by not over aggressively releasing the medial side upon the initial exposure (Figure 20-4).

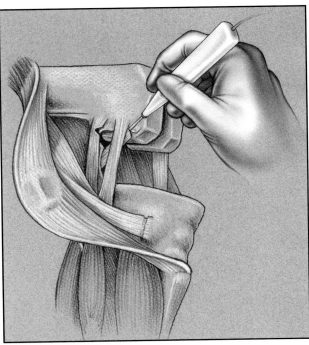

Figure 20-2. If the flexion space is not rectangular and the lateral side is tight, then the tight lateral structures are palpated and the tightest is released, which is usually the popliteus tendon. (Reproduced with permission of Joint Implant Surgeons, Inc.)

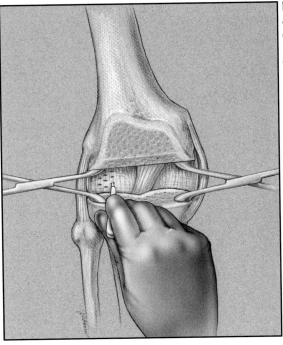

Figure 20-3. If the knee is still tight laterally, the laminar spreader is inserted in extension and the posterior capsule and lateral collateral ligament are lengthened through careful pie-crusting technique. (Reproduced with permission of Joint Implant Surgeons, Inc.)

Thus the routine order of releases includes the tightest structures first and proceeds through the next tightest structure until full extension is achieved, the joint space is rectangular in extension, and the joint space is rectangular in flexion. The most common order of releases would be: IT band, popliteus tendon, posterior capsule, LCL, and, rarely, the posterior-medial complex.

Figure 20-4. Avoid over aggressive release on the medial side upon the initial exposure, which may result in excessive opening of the joint space, elevation of the joint line, and strain on the peroneal nerve. (Reproduced with permission of Joint Implant Surgeons, Inc.)

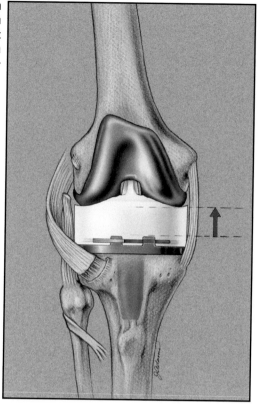

References

1. Buechel FF. A sequential three-step lateral release for correcting fixed valgus deformities during total knee arthroplasty. *Clin Orthop Relat Res*. 1990;260:170-175.
2. Insall JN, Easley ME. Surgical technique and instrumentation. In: Insall JN, Scott WN, eds. *Surgery of the Knee*. 3rd edition. Philadelphia: Churchill-Livingstone; 2001:1553-1620.
3. Krackow KA. Deformity. In: Krackow KA, ed. *The Technique of Total Knee Arthroplasty*. St. Louis, MO: Mosby; 1990:249-372.
4. Lombardi AV Jr. Total knee replacement: Valgus release. In: Cushner FD, Scott WN, Scuderi GR, eds. *Surgical Techniques for the Knee*. New York: Thieme Medical Publishers, Inc.; 2005:174-179.
5. Lombardi AV Jr, Dodds KL, Berend KR, Mallory TH, Adams JB. An algorithmic approach to valgus total knee arthroplasty. *J Bone Joint Surg Am*. 2004;86(Suppl 2):62-71.
6. Miyasaka KC, Ranawat CS, Mullaji A. 10- to 20-year follow-up of total knee arthroplasty for valgus deformities. *Clin Orthop Relat Res*. 1997;345:29-37.

IF I AM DOING A TOTAL KNEE AND IT IS TOO TIGHT IN EXTENSION, BUT OTHERWISE FEELS WELL BALANCED, WHAT SHOULD I DO?

Steven Stuchin, MD

Problems of total knee flexion extension balance can be considered in nine possible combinations (Table 21-1). The proximal tibia articulates with the posterior femur in flexion and the distal femur in extension. Changing the height of the proximal tibia by cutting more bone or changing the thickness of the polyethylene liner will change both flexion and extension gaps. Removing bone from the distal femur will affect only the extension gap (it will make it larger). Similarly, resecting more or less bone from the posterior aspect of the femur (eg, choosing a small or larger femoral component, respectively) will selectively effect the flexion gap.

If a knee is tight in flexion and extension (combination #1), decreasing the tibial height by cutting more bone or using a thinner polyethylene liner will increase the size of both gaps and if the gaps are symmetrically tight, the knee will now be balanced. Similarly, if a knee is loose in both flexion and extension (combination #5), a thicker polyethylene liner will tighten both gaps.

Combination #7, OK in flexion, tight in extension requires a solution that only affects the extension gap and may require some combination of soft tissue releases and bone cuts. Resecting more distal femur increases the extension gap without changing the flexion gap. Alternatively, if the patient had a preoperative flexion contracture, and the amount of bone resected from the distal femur is equivalent to the thickness of the prosthesis that is replacing it, then a posterior capsular release should be performed to increase the size of the extension gap. This includes not only releasing the posterior capsule from the posterior aspect of the femur but also removing any associated osteophytes that can tent the posterior capsule causing tightness in extension. Finally, if the tibia has been cut with a posterior slope, recutting at neutral will maintain the same balance in flexion, but will add a few degrees of extension.

Table 21-1

Problems of Total Knee Flexion Extension Balance

Combination	Flexion	Extension	Solution
1	Tight	Tight	Cut more tibia or thinner liner
2	Tight	Loose	Augment distal femur + thinner liner or downsize femur + thicker liner
3	Tight	OK	Release PCL, increase tibial slope or downsize femur
4	Loose	Tight	Solve as per 6
5	Loose	Loose	Thicker liner
6	Loose	OK	Upsize femur or thicker liner then solve as per 7
7	OK	Tight	Resect more distal femur or posterior release or decrease tibial slope
8	OK	Loose	Augment distal femur or downsize femur + thicker liner
9	OK	OK	OK

Combination #6, loose in flexion, OK in extension can be solved by either upsizing the femoral component or using a two-step solution. First, increase the polyethylene thickness; now the knee will be OK in flexion, but tight in extension (combination #7) so either resect more distal femur or perform a posterior capsular release. Combination #4 (loose in flexion and tight in extension) is a similar problem as #6, and has the same solution; upsize the femur and then either resect more distal femur or perform a posterior release or use a thicker liner followed by either increased distal femoral resection or a posterior release.

There are three combinations left to consider: 2, 3, and 8. If the knee is tight in flexion there are several potential solutions. If you are using a cruciate retaining knee the posterior cruciate ligament (PCL) can be resected to increase the flexion gap and then you can convert to a posterior stabilized (PS) total knee. Alternatively, the posterior slope of the tibial cut can be increased; this will also increase the size of the flexion gap. If you are able to partially correct the problem in 2 and 3 by increasing the flexion gap, then these problems resolve to #8 (OK in flexion, loose in extension), which is most easily fixed by augmenting the distal femur. Alternatively, combination #2 (tight in flexion, loose in extension) can be solved using distal augmentation on the femur combined with a thinner polyethylene liner.

If you are prepared to change the joint line (elevate it), then it is worth considering the use of an undersized femoral component as an alternative solution to fix a knee that is too tight in flexion. If the knee system you are using allows it, downsizing the femur will increase the flexion gap without changing the extension gap. This provides an alternative means of solving combination #8; using a thicker polyethylene liner with a downsized femur. In those circumstances where there is more than one solution, it is best to choose the option that best maintains the joint line.

Using a PS component is another way to solve some of these problems. The central post will allow for a few millimeters of flexion gap laxity. The tibial polyethylene liner can be decreased in thickness to increase the flexion and extension gaps. This may solve any of the combinations that allow for laxity in flexion. Combination #6 (loose in flexion, OK in extension) is the best example.

There are some authors who have suggested that residual flexion contracture may stretch out in therapy or that a lax knee will "tighten up" with time. Although this may happen on occasion, it is hardly predictable and most surgeons more likely see knees that were well executed go on to develop contracture in the ensuing weeks after surgery. Accordingly, the patient is best served when every effort is made to balance the knee at the time of surgery.

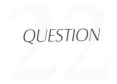
THE PATELLA MEASURES 22 MILLIMETERS PRIOR TO MAKING MY OSTEOTOMY. HOW MUCH BONE SHOULD I REMOVE?

Hari P. Bezwada, MD
Robert E. Booth, Jr., MD

The thickness of the native patella varies considerably, with females generally ranging from 20 to 25 mm and males from 23 to 28 mm. The absolute amount of bone resected in performing a patellar arthroplasty is therefore quite variable as well. One approach is to replace the patellar stature "1-for-1," and there are multiple resection tools and measurement devices to accomplish this goal.[1] The difficulty with this approach is that there is a relationship between the thickness of the patella and the configuration of the distal femur. In most male knees there is sufficient anterior femoral bone that will not be over-replaced by a standard femoral component. Thus, a "1-for-1" patellar replacement will not over stuff the anterior compartment of the knee, avoiding pain and restricted motion. In many other knees, most of which are female in gender, there is only a minimal amount of anterior femoral bone; and a standard femoral component will restore more thickness than was removed (Figure 22-1). Thus, a "1-for-1" patella replacement *will* over stuff the front of many total knee arthroplasties.

Although this ratio of femoral to patellar bone stock is incompletely understood by engineers and orthopedists, every knee has adapted to this condition. The junction between the intratendinous portion or body of the patella and the exposed dorsal surface or face of the patella is defined by the "patellar nose."[2] This prominence of the distal patella, incorporated into the patellar tendon and obscured by the infrapatellar fat pad, establishes a safe depth of patellar resection (Figure 22-2). If one identifies this sulcus, a saw blade cutting from tendon to tendon superiorly and from chondral surface to chondral surface transversely, will establish an appropriate resection for that particular knee (Figure 22-3).[3] The applied domical button, covering the exposed patellar surface from inferior to superior but rarely from medial to lateral, will create a composite that reliably measures roughly one millimeter less than the original natural patella. The patellar

Figure 22-1. Radiograph on left represents lateral view of a typical male knee; note build-up of anterior bone on the femur. Radiograph on the right represents a typical female knee; note the relative deficiency on anterior bone on the femur.

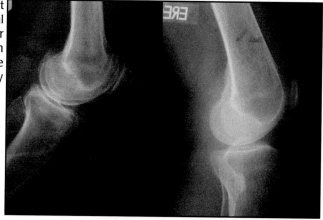

Figure 22-2. Close-up lateral radiograph of a knee demonstrating the patellar nose. The arrow points out the patellar nose, which represents the intratendinous portion of the patella.

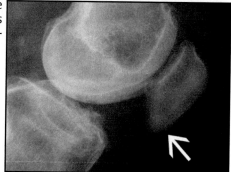

Figure 22-3. Intraoperative picture demonstrating the patellar resection utilizing the patellar nose as a guide to the level of resection.

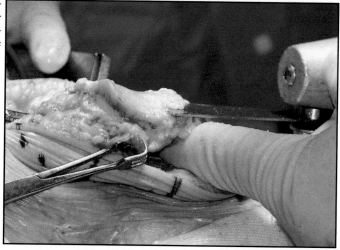

prosthesis, should, obviously, be placed on the medial and superior aspect of the cut patellar surface.

Under-resection or oblique resection of the patellar face will create an excessively thick patella, which will produce excessive tension in the anterior compartment of the knee. This may require a lateral retinacular release to improve tracking at the time of surgery. Worse, it may restrict flexion or produce anterior knee pain when negotiating stairs and chairs.

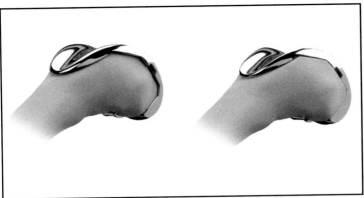

Figure 22-4. Pictures of the Gender Solutions Knee (Zimmer, Warsaw, IN). The male femoral component is pictured on the left and the female femoral component is pictured on the right. Note the thinner anterior flange on the female version along with less overhang.

Over-resection of the patella avoids overstuffing, but runs the risk of fracture or avascular necrosis. A residual patellar fragment of less than 12 mm has been shown to have compromised vascularity. Extensor mechanism ruptures are not uncommon after excessive patellar resection, and this is a very difficult complication to rectify.

In many female knees and a small percentage of male knees, pure patello-femoral arthritis is sufficiently severe to justify arthroplasty. In this setting, a conscious decompression of the anterior compartment of the knee would seem prudent, lest one recreate the same pathophysiology that prompted the surgery. In this setting, as well as in most female knees, the use of a gender-specific femoral component with a thinner femoral flange becomes a very attractive option (Figure 22-4). This construct allows the surgeon to perform a standard patellar resection—while avoiding excessive femoral replacement—in recreating the appropriate balance between femoral and patellar thickness.

References

1. Lachiewicz PF. Implant design and techniques for patellar resurfacing in total knee arthroplasty. *Instr Course Lect.* 2004;53:187-191.
2. Booth RE Jr. The patellar nose—an anatomic guide for patellar resurfacing; Coventry award presentation Knee Society Specialty Day; American Academy of Orthopaedic Surgeons; Orlando, Florida, 2000.
3. Lombardi AV Jr, Mallory TH, Maitino PD, Herrington SM, Kefauver CA. Freehand resection of the patella in total knee arthroplasty referencing the attachments of the quadriceps tendon and patella tendon. *J Arthroplasty.* 1998;13(7):788-792.

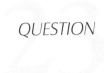

WHAT SHOULD I DO IF I CUT THE MCL INTRAOPERATIVELY?

Scott D. Ruhlman MD
Shanon M. Sara
Seth S. Leopold, MD

Injury to the medial collateral ligament (MCL) during total knee arthroplasty (TKA) is a known complication, occurring in 2.7 to 8% of patients in reported case series. The risk of iatrogenic injury to the MCL probably is increased in obese patients[1] or patients with previous osteotomies, in whom obtaining surgical exposure can be more difficult. MCL insufficiency after TKA can result in symptomatic instability and the need for revision arthroplasty.

MCL injuries occur during exposure, ligament balancing, femoral preparation, tibial preparation, and trial reduction. To avoid MCL injury, it is critical to see and protect the ligament during exposure. Careful retractor placement during bone cuts (keeping a retractor between the saw and the ligament) also helps prevent injury. If you remove the menisci, take care when you trim out the medial meniscus to observe and palpate the MCL (which is intimately apposed to the medial meniscus), so you don't inadvertently go too "wide" during meniscal excision and remove a band of the ligament along with the meniscal remnant. Finally, careful handling of the MCL in patients with osteoporosis, obesity, previous knee surgery, or chronic steroid use will decrease the likelihood of MCL injury.

Iatrogenic MCL injury historically has been treated with varus-valgus constrained implants, regardless of what the preoperative alignment had been. While such implants have satisfactory early- to mid-term results in difficult cases, the literature suggests that the additional constraint inherent in such designs increases stresses at the implant-cement and cement-bone interfaces, and therefore may predispose such implants to aseptic loosening. We therefore do not recommend using these implants where a less-constrained implant would work.

We studied the option of intraoperative repair or reattachment, combined with short-term use of a hinged knee brace, in TKAs where the MCL was iatrogenically injured. We found that stability was achieved without conversion to a constrained implant.[2] No patient required bracing beyond the 6-week postoperative period in this series, which included 16 primary MCL repairs at 45-month mean follow-up. There was no subjective instability, no demonstrable coronal-plane laxity on physical exam either at 30 degrees of flexion or in full extension, and no additional surgeries for treatment of the instability were required.[2] The patients in that series had neutral or varus alignment preoperatively; if the preoperative alignment is valgus, and the MCL is deficient or intraoperatively injured, we don't recommend simple repair. Rather, in that circumstance, we use a varus-valgus constrained implant; that is, an unlinked constrained device that includes a tall, reinforced tibial post and a deep femoral box. These implants should be inserted with stems, in order to transmit stresses generated by the constrained articulation away from the fixation interfaces at the joint line to more normal diaphyseal bone (cementless stems) or along a broader surface area of implant-cement bone contact (cemented stems). In this setting, these implants have good intermediate-term survival, although little is known about their performance beyond 10 years. Potential drawbacks of this approach, which we accept as necessary risks in the valgus knee, include increased bone-stock loss, potentially higher rates of aseptic loosening owing to increased constraint, fracture/failure of the tibial intercondylar eminence, and recurrent instability despite an intact intercondylar eminence.

Intraoperative MCL injuries occur as either midsubstance disruptions, avulsions of the ligament from the tibial insertion, or the femoral origin. For patients whose preoperative alignment was neutral or varus, we would employ the following techniques for the management of intraoperative MCL injury during TKA:

1. For midsubstance disruptions, we would consider using a running, locking (eg, modified Krackow), nonabsorbable suture with direct end-to-end repair (Figure 23-1).

2. For distal avulsions, we would consider using either suture anchors or a repair tied over a screw-post. Suturing of these avulsions usually can again be done with the modified Krackow stitch (running, locking suture). If suture anchors are not used, reinforcement with a spiked washer and a screw sometimes is possible (Figures 23-2 and 23-3).

3. For proximal avulsions, a large screw with a spiked washer is often satisfactory, as these usually present as epicondylar avulsions in osteopenic bone.

Regardless of the location of the injury, we recommend performing the repair or reattachment prior to cementing the final components, and tensioning the repair in slight- to mid-flexion with the appropriate thickness polyethylene trial in place; be sure to verify that excellent ligament balance is present in both extension and flexion, and to test stability and range of motion.

Postoperatively, we would allow full weight bearing in a hinged knee brace for 6 weeks, free range of motion, and in all other respects, routine aftercare.

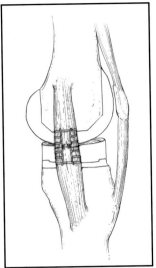 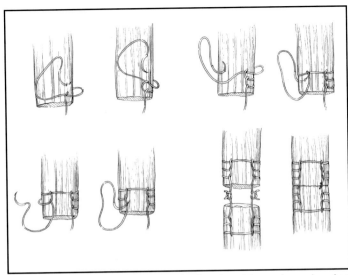

Figure 23-1. Diagram showing intrasubstance repair of MCL with direct end-to-end repair using four strands of a running, locking, nonabsorbable, braided suture.

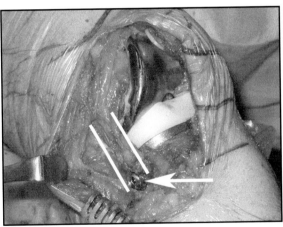

Figure 23-2. Intraoperative appearance following repair of an MCL avulsion using a screw and washer (arrow). The MCL has been outlined with solid white lines.

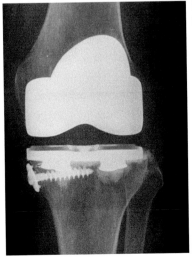

Figure 23-3. Postoperative radiograph showing the screw and washer.

References

1. Winiarsky R, Barth P, Lotke P. Total knee arthroplasty in morbidly obese patients. *J Bone Joint Surg Am.* 1998; 80-A:1770-1774.
2. Leopold SS, McStay C, Klafeta K, Jacobs JJ, Berger RA, Rosenberg AG. Primary repair of intraoperative disruption of the medial collateral ligament during total knee arthroplasty. *J Bone Joint Surg Am.* 2001;83-A:86-91.

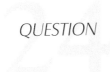

WHEN DO YOU USE ANTIBIOTIC-LOADED CEMENT?

Mohammad Namazian, DO
Paul E. Di Cesare, MD

The concept of cement as an antibiotic depot, introduced in the 1970s, has become an integral part of the treatment and prophylaxis of musculoskeletal infections, especially in the prevention and treatment of infections involving total joint arthroplasty (TJA).

Indications

Antibiotic-impregnated cement in TJA can be used for definitive fixation of implants or as a temporary spacer for the resolution of a documented infection. In the former case it is indicated for primary joint replacement with or without a history of resolved infection at the operative site, including patients with no history of infection or previous surgery, those with a history of resolved previous joint or arthroplasty infection, those with retained implants at the site of a previous joint surgery, and those who have undergone a two-stage exchange for infection and are now undergoing the final reimplantation. The routine use of antibiotic-impregnated cement in uncomplicated primary TJA remains controversial, as some cite the potential increased resistance of infecting bacteria and others argue that the risk must be weighed against the lower reported infection rates of arthroplasties implanted with antibiotic cement.[1] The routine use of antibiotic-impregnated cement in patients that are more prone to infection due to systemic disease such as diabetes mellitus and rheumatoid arthritis is strongly recommended.

Antibiotic-impregnated cement as a temporary spacer is indicated for two-stage exchange procedures of infected TJA. In resection arthroplasty for infection it provides the following advantages: (1) delivers high concentrations of antibiotics locally without systemic side effects; (2) maintains joint height and limb length; (3) retains joint mobil-

Table 24-1

FDA-Approved Premixed Antibiotic-Impregnated Cements

Name	Manufacturer	Antibiotic per 40 g of Cement
VersaBond AB	Smith & Nephew	1.0 g Gentamicin
Simplex P	Stryker	1.0 g Tobramycin
Cemex Genta	Exactech	0.5 g Gentamicin
Palacos G	Zimmer	0.5 g Gentamicin
Cobalt G-HV	Biomet	0.5 g Tobramycin
Cobalt G-HV	DePuy Orthopaedics	1.0 g Gentamicin

Note: FDA approval is only for implantation at the site of a two-stage exchange procedure.

ity and stability, especially when articulating spacers are used; (4) diminishes soft tissue contractures; and (5) facilitates ease of reimplantation.

Antibiotic-impregnated beads of cement on a string can be utilized as a treatment adjunct in acutely infected total joints; beads are placed about the joint at the time of irrigation and debridement and removed shortly thereafter.

Preparation

Antibiotic-impregnated cement for definitive implantation of prosthetic devices can be hand-mixed in the operating room or purchased premixed (Table 24-1). The advantages of hand-mixing include lower cost and the ability to customize antibiotic choice and dose. The ratio of antibiotics to cement influences the mechanical properties of cured cement. The current consensus is to use 1 to 2 g antibiotic per 40-g package of bone cement for final implantation in TJA. The choice of antibiotic also affects the volume that can be used safely without altering its mechanical properties of cement. Persson et al reported that the mechanical properties of cement are altered by addition of 2.5% of vancomycin but not by 1.25% of vancomycin nor 1.25% of meropenem. This is thought to be due to the amphoteric properties of vancomycin, resulting in a lower-molecular-weight polymetric chain that compromises the mechanical properties of cement.

Hand-mixing is optimized by utilizing a small mesh strainer to obtain an ultrafine powder.[2] Vacuum-mixing also improves the mechanical properties of antibiotic cement. Postak and Greenwald nevertheless reported that the mechanical properties of hand-mixed cement are inferior to the premixed form.[3]

A recent study has confirmed that species of staphylococcus, streptococcus, and enterococcus account for the majority of periprosthetic infections, with sensitivity profiles of 96% to vancomycin, 90% to tobramycin, and 88% to gentamicin.[4] Elusion characteristics

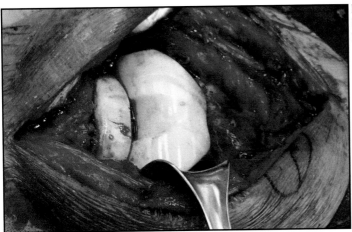

Figure 24-1. InterSpace articulating antibiotic impregnated knee spacer (Exactech).

of antibiotics from bone cement also vary depending on brand; Palacos bone cement has been reported to provide higher elusion levels than others.[5,6]

The current standard of care for a chronic periprosthetic joint infection is a two-stage revision with use of a temporary antibiotic-impregnated cement spacer between stages. Spacers can be prepared in the operating room or purchased prefabricated and can be either static or articulating. Prefabricated articulating spacers for the knee include the Prostalac system (DePuy) and the InterSpace system (Exactech, Gainesville, FL) (Figure 24-1). Operating room preparation involves using no more than 8 g antibiotic per 40-g pack of bone cement as higher concentrations will adversely affect the curing and handling process.[7] Also, additional monomer solution should be used and titrated based on quantity of antibiotic used. Choice of antibiotic should be guided by cultures obtained prior to explanation. If cultures fail to identify an organism, coverage should include vancomycin or tobramycin, which cover 90% of potential infecting organisms.

Precautions

High-dose antibiotic-impregnated cement spacers for two-stage exchange of infected total hip arthroplasty have been associated with acute renal failure, which can take several months to develop and in all reported cases resolved with extraction of the spacer. Allergic reaction to the antibiotic in the spacer has rarely occurred.

Conclusion

Antibiotic-impregnated cement provides a method of delivering high concentrations of antibiotics locally to an infected site over an extended period of time without overt adverse systemic effects. Because the mechanical properties of bone cement are altered by the addition of antibiotics, concentration and choice of antibiotics need to reflect the specific needs of the patient.

References

1. Engesaeter LB, Espehaug B, Lie AS, Furnes O, Havenlin LI. Does cement increase the risk of infection in primary total hip arthroplasty? *Acta Orthopaedica*. 2006;77(3):351-358.
2. Krackaw KA, Rauh MA, Meredith RM, Munjal S. Antibiotic-laden cement. *J Arthroplasty*. 2005;20(7):941-942.
3. Postak PD, Greenwald AS. The influence of antibiotics on the fatigue life of acrylic bone cement. *J Bone Joint Surgery*. 2006;88-A(Supp 4):148-155.
4 Fulkerson E, Della Valle CJ, Wise B, Walsh M, Preston C, Di Cesare PE. Antibiotic susceptibility of bacteria infecting TJA sites. *J Bone Joint Surgery*. 2006;88-A(6):1231-1237.
5. Penner MJ, Duncam CP, Masri BA. The in vitro elusion characteristics of antibiotics-loaded CMV and Palacos-R bone cement. *J Arthroplasty*. 1999;14:209-214.
6. Kuechle DK, Landon GC, Musher DM, Nobel PC. Elusion of vancomycin, daptomycin, and amikacin from acrylic bone cement. *Clin Orthop*. 1999;264:302-308.
7. Hsieh PH, Chang YH, Chen SH, Ueng SW, Shih CH. High concentrations and bioactivity of vancomycin and aztreonam elude from simplex cement spacers in two-stage revision of infected hip implants: A study of 46 patients at an average follow-up of 107 days. *J Orthopedic Res*. 2006 Aug;1615-1621.

Do You Inject the Capsule With Anything at the End of the Case in an Effort to Decrease Perioperative Pain?

Amanda Marshall, MD

The goals of postoperative pain management are to not only facilitate rehab and early return to normal function, but to satisfy our humanitarian obligation to minimize the patient's pain. Meeting these goals translates into improved patient satisfaction. In recent years, surgeons have become increasingly aware of the complications caused by under treated acute pain following total knee arthroplasty. The trend is to take a multimodal approach to treating such perioperative pain. One facet of this approach consists of an injection of various substances into the periarticular tissues at the time of surgery.

The objective of the injection is to target both peripheral and central sensitization that occurs at the time of the surgical trauma. Centrally, the input is via heightened excitability of the spinal neurons and presence of opioid receptors within the local tissues. The opioid receptors are expressed within hours postoperatively and have afferent sensory input to the CNS. Peripherally, the sensitivity of the nociceptive neurons is increased. This in conjunction with increased levels of inflammatory mediators heightens the pain response. The goal of the common ingredients found in the periarticular injections (which include opioids, anti-inflammatory drugs, and local anesthetic agents) is to block these various pathways.

I routinely use a cocktail consisting of 15 mg of Toradol (0.5 mL of 30 mg/mL ketorolac), 150 mg bupivacaine (20 mL of 0.75%), 2 mg morphine (2 mL of 1 mg/mL Duramorph-preservative free), and 0.3 mg epinephrine (0.3 mL of 1 mg/mL 1:1000) combined with normal saline for a combined volume of 60 cc. This is prepared the morning of the case in the pharmacy. The first 20 mL is injected into the posterior capsule and the medial and lateral collateral ligaments prior to placing the polyethylene insert. It is imperative to avoid injecting too near the common peroneal nerve. The remaining solution is injected in the retinacular tissues, extensor mechanism, and subcuticular areas prior to closure.

My method is similar to that of other authors[1-3] with the primary difference being the various dosages of medications. Busch et al utilize a 100 mL solution consisting of 400 mg of ropivicaine, 30 mg of Toradol, 5 mg of epimorphine, and 0.6 mL of epinephrine (1:1000) in normal saline. The injection sites are also similar with 20 mL injected posteriorly, 20 mL in the extensor mechanism/retinaculum, and 60 mL in the fat and subcuticular tissues. Lombardi et al advocated a combined soft tissue injection with an intra-articular injection. His technique consists of bupivacaine and epinephrine in the muscle and synovium and another injection with bupivacaine, epinephrine, and morphine in the joint following capsular closure.

The few studies available all reveal decreased pain scores in the immediate postoperative period compared to control groups. In addition, the need for supplemental analgesia is also reduced. Lombardi's study also demonstrated a lower bleeding index and overall blood loss for the injection group. No cardiac or central nervous system complications have been observed in any of the studies. A recent study by Deirmengian et al examined the level of bupivacaine in the reinfusion drain after a periarticular injection. The bupivacaine levels both in the drain and in the serum postreinfusion were far below the toxic serum threshold. The total bupivacaine in the reinfusion blood was only 1% of the total bupivacaine used as the local anesthetic.

Overall, multimodal pain management protocols are resulting in better patient satisfaction and less postoperative pain. The periarticular injection is one of the tools in our armamentarium to better facilitate improved patient outcomes following total knee arthroplasty.

References

1. Busch CA, Shore BJ, Bhandari R, Ganapathy S, MacDonald SJ, Bourne RB, Rorabeck CH, McCalden RW. Efficacy of periarticular multimodal drug injection in total knee arthroplasty—a randomized trial. *JBJS—Am.* 2006;88:959-963.
2. Lombardi AV, Berend KR, Mallory TH, Dodds KL, Adams JB. Soft tissue and intraarticular injection of bupivacaine, epinephrine, and morphine has a beneficial effect after total knee arthroplasty. *CORR.* 2004;428:125-130.
3. Ranawat CS. Controlling pain after total hip and knee replacement using a multimodal protocol with local periarticular injections: a prospective randomized study. Hip Society Meeting, 2007.
4. Marshall AD, Masonis JL, Mokris JG, Oesterle JR, Camp J, Mauerhan DR. Postoperative pain following total knee arthroplasty: A prospective, double-blinded, randomized study comparing IV patient-controlled-analgesia, pericapsular knee injection, and femoral nerve block. AAHKS Meeting, 2005.
5. Deirmengian CA, Abella L, Paprosky WG, Sporer SM. Bupivacaine levels in the reinfusion drain after periarticular injection during TKA. AAOS Meeting, 2007.

SECTION III

POSTOPERATIVE QUESTIONS

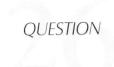

I HAVE A PATIENT WHO IS 2 WEEKS POSTOPERATIVE FROM A PRIMARY TOTAL KNEE ARTHROPLASTY AND THE WOUND IS DRAINING. WHAT SHOULD I DO?

Carl Deirmengian, MD

The concern over any persistently draining wound after total knee arthroplasty (TKA) is the possibility of deep infection. It is normal to have some drainage from the incision after hip or knee arthroplasty. In a retrospective study of 2,437 consecutive hip and knee arthroplasties,[1] it was found that most patients drain for a few days postoperatively. By day 3 after surgery, approximately 50% of patients still had some drainage, but by day 5 to 6, almost all patients have a dry incision. Once the drainage persists into the second week after surgery, serious concern should exist regarding the risk of postoperative infection.

Some instances of persistent drainage at 2 weeks are clearly deep infections (associated with systemic systems such as fever or grossly purulent drainage) and should be returned to the OR for an irrigation and debridement with exchange of the polyethylene liner. Multiple deep cultures are sent prior to the administration of antibiotics, in order to identify the infecting organism and tailor the antibiotic regimen. Intravenous antibiotics are then administered for 6 weeks in conjunction with an infectious disease specialist, and in some cases an oral antibiotic is continued for several months after the intravenous antibiotics are finished depending on organism sensitivity, the status of the host, and the infectious disease specialist's recommendations. In a retrospective study of 546 primary and 51 revision TKAs,[2] early irrigation and debridement was indicated in 8 patients for persistent wound drainage. Two patients had positive synovial fluid cultures and were treated successfully with a 6-week course of intravenous antibiotics.

Other cases of drainage 2 weeks after TKA are clearly not deep infections, but rather represent delayed, superficial wound healing issues that produce scant drainage in the setting of an otherwise benign knee. These patients progress otherwise normally after surgery, but should be monitored closely for improvement and ultimate healing. Antibiotics should not be administered unless a synovial fluid aspirate has been obtained to rule out the presence of deep infection. There is some evidence[3] to suggest that in the absence of deep infection, early surgical intervention for these patients may lead to a higher rate of major subsequent surgery and/or deep infection.

Unfortunately, the history and physical examination of a patient with drainage at 2 weeks postoperatively oftentimes does not lead to a definitive diagnosis, and you are faced with a clinical dilemma. A patient may present with no systemic symptoms, a mild effusion, pain that appears typical for 2 weeks postoperatively and persistent, nonpurulent drainage.

The c-reactive protein (CRP), erythrocyte sedimentation rate (ESR), and imaging studies will be nonspecific 2 weeks postoperatively. The only useful diagnostic tool remaining is an aspiration of the synovial fluid. A culture can be sent that may identify bacterial growth, and a synovial fluid white blood cell (wbc) count with differential is obtained.

After sending a wbc count and culture, there are two possible results that would push most surgeons to proceed with an early irrigation and debridement. For one, positive synovial fluid cultures or a gram stain that shows the presence of organisms would be diagnostic for acute postoperative infection. Secondly, a high synovial fluid wbc count would be diagnostic for infection. Although there are studies that have examined the utility of the synovial fluid wbc to identify infection at the site of a TKA, little data is available to determine the utility of this test in the early postoperative period. Certainly if the wbc count is greater than 20,000 cells/mm^3, most surgeons would make the diagnosis of infection and proceed with operative debridement. However it is difficult to interpret mildly elevated cell counts in the range of 2000 to 20,000 cells/mm^3 because of the likely presence of inflammation and hematoma remaining after TKA. In such equivocal cases, it is reasonable to start oral antibiotics, continue watching the cultures, and closely monitor the wound. Oral antibiotics are given for the duration of drainage in an attempt to prevent bacterial seeding of the joint.

However, if the drainage does not appear to be decreasing at 2 weeks an exploratory debridement is indicated. The wound is incised and the source of drainage is explored. Oftentimes, a defect in the arthrotomy is discovered and if any communication beyond the retinaculum is identified, a complete irrigation and debridement with polyethylene change is necessary.

The management of persistent drainage 2 weeks after TKA is difficult; however, the liberal use of synovial fluid aspiration can assist the surgeon in identifying cases of deep infection that require irrigation and debridement.

References

1. Patel VP, Walsh M, Sehgal B, Preston C, DeWal H, Di Cesare PE. Factors associated with prolonged wound drainage after primary total hip and knee arthroplasty. *J Bone Joint Surg Am.* 2007 Jan;89(1):33-38.
2. Weiss AP, Krackow KA. Persistent wound drainage after primary total knee arthroplasty. *J Arthroplasty.* 1993 Jun;8(3):285-289.
3. Galat DD, McGovern SC, Hanssen AD, Clarke HD. Surgical treatment of early wound complications after primary total knee arthroplasty. *J Arthroplasty.* 22(2):313-322.

WHAT IS THE BEST METHOD FOR PREVENTING THROMBOEMBOLIC EVENTS AFTER TOTAL KNEE ARTHROPLASTY?

Jay R. Lieberman, MD

Total knee arthroplasty is an extremely successful operation that relieves pain, improves function, and enhances the quality of patients' lives. However, patients who have a total knee arthroplasty are at risk for the development of venous thromboembolic disease. Therefore, it is essential that an effective method of prophylaxis be selected for patients undergoing total knee arthroplasty.

In North America, there is general agreement that deep vein thrombosis (DVT) prophylaxis is necessary after total knee arthroplasty but the ideal prophylactic regimen has not been identified. The selection of a prophylaxis regimen involves a balance between efficacy and safety. Surgeons are particularly concerned about bleeding after total knee arthroplasty because it can lead to hematoma formation, infection, reoperation, and a prolonged hospital stay. Hematoma can lead to stiffness and reduce the postoperative range of motion, which can have a negative impact on the patient's overall outcome. The selection of a prophylaxis agent is also influenced by the more frequent use of regional anesthesia, the development of perioperative pain protocols that include anti-inflammatory medications that may also increase the risk of bleeding, and the continued decrease in the duration of hospital stays. Over the past decade a number of agents have been found to provide safe and effective DVT prophylaxis after total knee arthroplasty.[1]

The overall rates of DVT are higher after total knee arthroplasty then after total hip arthroplasty; however, the rates of symptomatic pulmonary embolism are higher after total hip replacement. Both pharmacologic agents and mechanical devices provide safe and effective prophylaxis after total knee arthroplasty.

Pharmacologic Methods

WARFARIN

Warfarin has been used successfully as a prophylaxis agent following total knee arthroplasty for approximately 30 years. Warfarin inhibits the production of the vitamin K dependent clotting factors II, VII, IX, and X in the liver. Warfarin has been shown in both randomized trials and cohort studies to provide safe and effective prophylaxis after total knee arthroplasty. The major advantage of warfarin is that it is an oral agent. Warfarin like other pharmacologic agents is associated with bleeding but the bleeding risk is actually low if the INR can be maintained at the appropriate level. However, the use of warfarin has several disadvantages. First, regular monitoring of the international normalized ratio (INR) is necessary. The target INR should be 2.0. Second, warfarin is started the evening of the day of the surgery but the drug has a delayed onset of action and there is concern that patients may be relatively unprotected from either the development of a blood clot or its propagation during the early postoperative period. Third, warfarin interacts with numerous medications because it is metabolized in the cytochrome P450 system in the liver. Because warfarin has a delayed onset of action it is strongly recommended that the drug be continued after hospital discharge.[1]

In randomized trials warfarin was not as efficacious as the low molecular weight heparins in limiting the formation of asymptomatic clots (proximal clot rates were 10 to 12% for warfarin and 0 to 8% for LMWHs). However, there was a general trend toward decreased bleeding rates with warfarin use.

LOW MOLECULAR WEIGHT HEPARIN

Low molecular weight heparins (LMWH) generally have a molecular weight between 1000 and 10,000 Da. These LMWHs are prepared by either chemical or enzymatic depolymerization of unfractionated heparin. The antithrombotic activity of LMWH is via inhibition of the formation of factor Xa. Because of their molecular size the low molecular weight heparins are able to inhibit factor Xa but not thrombin.

The major advantages of use of the low molecular weight heparin are that there is good bioavailability and no monitoring is required. In general, a fixed dose of LMWH can be used. The LMWHs are metabolized in the kidney and therefore these agents must be used with caution in patients with renal insufficiency. The major disadvantages of the use of the LMWHs are that it requires parenteral administration and there are concerns about increased bleeding rates and wound drainage. The LMWHs have been associated with epidural bleeding. Guidelines have now been set forth to limit this bleeding risk. These guidelines include the following: an indwelling catheter should be removed prior to initiation of LMWH; the first dose of LMWH should be delayed 2 hours after catheter removal; when using a continuous epidural catheter the catheter removal should be delayed ten to twelve hours after the last dose of LMWH.[2]

The dosing regimens of the two most popular low molecular weight heparins used in North America, enoxaparin and dalteparin, are different. It is recommended that the initial dose of enoxaparin be administered 12 to 24 hours after the end of the surgical procedure. In contrast, a half dose of dalteparin is usually given approximately 4 hours after the operative procedure and then the patient receives the full dose on the first postoperative day. Overall the LMWHs provide both effective and safe prophylaxis after total knee arthroplasty.[3]

FONDAPARINUX

Fondaparinux is a synthetic pentasaccharide that acts as a specific inhibitor of factor Xa. The Fondaparinux selectively binds to anti-thrombin III, which results in an irreversible conformational change in the binding site for the factor Xa. There is no direct inhibition of thrombin. Fondaparinux is administered via a once daily parenteral dose (2.5 mg per day). It has been shown to provide safe and effective prophylaxis after total knee arthroplasty. In a randomized trial comparing fondaparinux to the LMWH enoxaparin, fondaparinux was more effective in preventing overall thrombus formation (12.5% vs 27.8%, p < .001). However, there were 11 major bleeding episodes in the fondaparinux group and there was one major bleed episode in the enoxaparin group. The advantage of this agent is that no monitoring is required and it is administered once per day. The major disadvantage is that it may be associated with higher bleeding rates and thrombocytopenia. Fondaparinux is also metabolized in the kidney and must be used judiciously in patients with renal failure.[4]

ASPIRIN

Aspirin limits platelet aggregation by inhibiting thromoxane A2 and the hypothesis is that this decreases thrombus formation. The advantages of aspirin are that it is an oral anti-platelet agent, no monitoring is required, and the bleeding rates are low. Aspirin has not been analyzed extensively in randomized trials using either venograms as an endpoint or symptomatic events. Aspirin has been evaluated in some small single center studies that revealed mechanical devices alone provided effective prophylaxis and no additional benefit was obtained with aspirin prophylaxis. Aspirin seems to reduce the overall rate of symptomatic venous thromboembolic disease after total knee arthroplasty but does not appear to be as effective as LMWH, warfarin, or mechanical devices. Knee surgeons often use aspirin combined with mechanical devices but the potential benefits of stacking modalities has not been determined in randomized trials.[1]

Mechanical Methods

Pneumatic compression boots (PCB) reduce stasis in the lower extremity by increasing the velocity of venous blood flow and by the enhancement of local endogenous fibrinolytic activity. Intermittent plantar compression of the foot is another form of mechanical prophylaxis. These devices mimic the hemodynamic effects that are noted during normal walking and theoretically this leads to an enhancement of venous return. The advantages of these two types of mechanical prophylaxis are that no laboratory monitoring is required and there is no risk of bleeding. Another advantage of intermittent plantar compression (IPC) is that the device is just worn on the foot and it is better tolerated by patients. The major disadvantage of both of these mechanical devices is that prophylaxis ceases at the time of hospital discharge. This may have a critical effect on efficacy when hospital stays have been reduced to 3 days or less for many total knee arthroplasty patients. In addition, another major problem is compliance. The patients do not receive any prophylaxis if they are not wearing the devices. This is one of the major reasons why surgeons like to use these devices in conjunction with other agents.

Pneumatic compression boots have been demonstrated to be efficacious in a number of single center randomized trials. The overall DVT rate in these studies varied from 20 to 38% and the proximal clot rates were only 7%. It is important to note that these were small studies and only 110 patients were studied. Intermittent plantar compression has also been analyzed in four studies. The overall risk reduction in these studies was 37% but again there was only a limited number of patients studied (172 patients). In two of the studies a LMWH was more effective than intermittent plantar compression reducing the overall DVT rate.[1]

On the basis of these studies both PCB and IPC appear to reduce DVT rates after total knee arthroplasty. The true efficacy of these agents needs to be studied in large multi-center randomized trials. As stated previously surgeons have been stacking modalities because warfarin has a delayed onset of action and a full dose LMWH is not received until the day after surgery. It has not been determined if a combination of a chemoprophylactic agent and a mechanical device provides additional protection for patients.[1]

DURATION OF PROPHYLAXIS

There is no data at the present time to support the use of extended duration prophylaxis after total knee arthroplasty. Two weeks of prophylaxis should be adequate for most total knee arthroplasty patients. Prolonged prophylaxis should be considered for patients with a history of venous thromboembolic disease or other risk factors such as limited mobilization. Routine screening has not been shown to be cost effective.

Recommendations

Total knee arthroplasty is a very successful operation that can enhance function and reduce pain. Patients who undergo these procedures are at increased risk for the development of pulmonary embolism and DVT. The most effective prophylactic agents for these patients include LMWH, warfarin, and fondaparinux. Aspirin appears to reduce the risk of symptomatic events but further study of this agent is necessary. Mechanical devices provide effective prophylaxis after total knee arthroplasty but further studies are necessary to determine their efficacy because hospital stays have been reduced over the past 5 years. Recently, the Centers for Medicare and Medicaid services have made recommendations regarding prophylaxis after total knee arthroplasty. The recommended agents included warfarin, LMWH, fondaparinux, and pneumatic compression boots. We are still seeking the ideal prophylactic regimen. This regimen would be an oral agent that requires no monitoring and has a low bleeding rate.

References

1. Lieberman JR, Wellington HSU. Prevention of venous thromboembolic disease after total hip and knee arthroplasty. *J Bone Joint Surg Am.* 2005;87:2097-2112.
2. Horlocker TT, Wedel DJ, Benzon H, Brown DL, Enneking FK, Heit JA, Mulroy MF, Rosenquist RW, Rowlingson J, Tryba M, Yuan CS. Regional anesthesia in the anticoagulated patient: defining the risks. *Reg Anesth Pain Med.* 2003;28:172-197.
3. Whang PG, Lieberman JR. Low-molecular-weight heparin. *J Am Acad Orthop Surg.* 2002;10:299-302.
4. Bauer KA, Eriksson BI, Lassen MR, Turpie AG. Steering Committee of the Pentasaccharide in Major Knee Surgery Study. Fondaparinux compared with enoxaparin for the prevention of venous thromboembolism after elective major knee surgery. *N Engl J Med.* 2001;345:1305-1310.

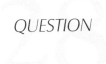

In the Recovery Room My Patient Does Not Have a Distal Pulse in the Operative Leg. What Should I Do?

Kevin B. Fricka, MD

Vascular injury after total knee arthroplasty (TKA) is rare (incidence between 0.03 and 0.17%) and the evaluation and management may be unfamiliar to the orthopaedic surgeon.[1,4] However, a delay in diagnosis and treatment can be disastrous, with morbidity that includes compartment syndrome and associated peroneal nerve palsy, wound healing problems, deep infection, and potential loss of limb; in prior reports, the amputation rate has ranged from 25% to 70%.[1-4]

If discovered in the recovery room, remove all compressive dressings and perform a careful physical exam to identify a dorsalis pedis and/or posterior tibial pulse. If these are not clearly palpable, perform a doppler exam; if distal flow is not identified, a vascular surgery consultation is immediately obtained. It is often difficult to assess signs of arterial occlusion or diminished vascular flow (pallor, poor/absent capillary refill, pain, paresthesias, and paralysis) without fully exposing the extremity. With the more frequent use of regional anesthetic, signs of pain and paresthesias can be attributed to the epidural or masked by the spinal anesthetic leading to a delay in diagnosis.

At our institution, the vascular surgeon will attempt to measure the ankle-brachial index (ABI) to determine the presence and degree of ischemia, and the use of angiogram will be time and setting dependent. If an intraoperative vascular suite is available, the angiogram does not need to be completed prior to returning to the operating room (OR). Similarly, if the ischemia time is prolonged before diagnosis, an angiogram is deferred in order to shorten the time to revascularization.

Intraoperative bleeding complications discovered after torniquet release are best evaluated with a direct vascular surgery consultation obtained in the OR. Most vascular complications, however, are discovered postoperatively and aggressive revascularization is essential to achieve limb salvage. Attempts at simple thrombectomy alone are routinely not sufficient and restoration of flow with bypass grafts (preferentially the contralateral greater saphenous vein) is usually indicated. To avoid associated complications, the liberal use of fasciotomies is recommended.

Understanding the risk factors for arterial complications after TKA can help the surgeon decrease the morbidity associated with this by encouraging a comprehensive preoperative vascular exam, with vascular surgery referral if indicated, and expeditious postoperative recognition. Patient risk factors include a history of arterial insufficiency including intermittent claudication, rest pain, a history of lower extremity ulcerations, previous vascular surgery, and absent or asymmetrical pulses. The presence of a popliteal mass may represent a popliteal aneurysm, which can be distinguished from a baker's cyst by ultrasound or the presence of a palpable or audible bruit; this should be repaired prior to undertaking TKA. The presence of radiographic vascular calcifications is an objective finding consistent with a history of peripheral vascular disease and Question 4 deals with the use of tourniquets in this setting. An ankle brachial index (ABI) of less than 0.9 is a risk factor for arterial complications and I routinely send these patients for a vascular surgery consultation to clarify the risks of TKA to the patient. An ABI of less than 0.5 mandates an angiogram as immediate revascularization may be necessary prior to TKA. Surgical risk factors for vascular injury include revision TKA, correction of severe deformity (especially flexion contractures), and the use of a tourniquet.

Vascular complications after TKA can be classified into four general types: arterial occlusion, arterial severance, arteriovenous fistula formation, and arterial aneurysm formation. The most common mechanism is probably arterial occlusion related to low flow from tourniquet use and manipulation of the popliteal artery during surgery, which leads to thrombosis. The majority of patients seeking knee arthroplasty have some degree of atherosclerotic plaque formation, which decreases the elasticity of the vessels and therefore can result in distortion, traction, and fracture of the plaque when the knee is manipulated or a tourniquet is inflated.

Anatomical MRI studies confirm the lateral positioning of the popliteal artery in relation to the posterior cruciate ligament (PCL) both at the level of the joint line and at the level of tibial and femoral resection.[3] Careful placement of retractors can help avoid direct injury (ie, I use either a double pronged retractor that straddles the PCL or a single prong retractor placed medial to the PCL). Avoid excessive hyperextension after all bone cuts are completed (such as lifting the extended and unsupported limb for any reason) as this places the artery under severe stretch over the sharp posterior edge of the tibia.

Prior to surgery, I know the pulse status of the limb. Some have suggested routine deflation of the tourniquet prior to polyethylene insertion to assess for hemorrhagic vascular complications. However, my routine consists of tourniquet deflation after closure and examination of the patient's posterior tibialis and dorsalis pedal pulses at the end of surgery with the patient still under anesthesia. This should be adopted as part of the surgical routine to minimize delays in diagnosis.

References

1. Calligaro KD, Dougherty MJ, Ryan S, Booth RE. Acute arterial complications associated with total hip and knee arthroplasty. *J Vasc Surg.* 2003;38:1170-1177.
2. Kumar SN, Chapman JA, Rawlins I. Vascular injuries in total knee arthroplasty: a review of the problem with special reference to the tourniquet. *J Arthroplasty.* 1998;13:211-216.
3. Ninomiya JT, Dean JC, Goldberg VM. Injury to the popliteal artery and its anatomic location in total knee arthroplasty. *J Arthroplasty.* 1999;14:803-809.
4. Rand JA. Vascular complications of total knee arthroplasty. *J Arthroplasty.* 1987;2:89-93.

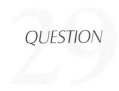

MY PATIENT HAS A FOOT-DROP AFTER SURGERY. WHAT SHOULD I DO?

Mark F. Schinsky, MD
William Macaulay, MD

Peripheral nerve palsy after total knee arthroplasty (TKA) is a rare and often unexpected complication. The reported incidence varies depending on the complexity of the specific patient population, implants used, specific nerve involvement, size of the study, method of diagnosis, and surgeon experience.[1] In our recent study and other large (>1,000 patients) reviews of consecutive TKAs, the incidence has ranged from 0.3% to 1.3%.[1,2]

Neurologic impairment following TKA typically involves the peroneal nerve. The peroneal nerve enters the popliteal space posteriorly then courses lateral to the fibular head. At the level of the fibular head, the nerve is superficial and particularly susceptible to compression. Peroneal neuropathy can lead to decreased sensation over the dorsum of the foot and ankle and loss of motor function, commonly referred to as a *foot-drop*. When tibial neuropathy is present, foot plantar flexion and inversion is weakened or absent, and sensation to the plantar aspect of the foot can be impaired or lost. We have found that dysesthesias and other pain syndromes associated with a peroneal nerve injury can be even more problematic for the patient than the loss of sensation and/or motor impairment.

Several factors have been associated with the development of peroneal nerve palsy after TKA including severe valgus and/or flexion contractures, preexisting neuropathy resulting from entities such as diabetes mellitus, alcoholism, or a more proximal nerve lesion (such as lumbar stenosis), rheumatoid arthritis, postoperative epidural analgesia, prolonged tourniquet use, external leg compression, and/or hematoma formation.[3-6] Patients with a preexisting risk factor should be educated preoperatively that they are potentially at higher risk for a peroneal nerve palsy.

Once a peroneal nerve palsy has been identified postoperatively, we recommend the removal of all potentially constrictive dressings and repositioning the knee in 25 to 40 degrees of flexion. This action relieves extrinsic compression from the dressings and

Figure 29-1. Exposed peroneal nerve during decompression as it travels from the popliteal space posteriorly to a more superficial and lateral position around the fibular head.

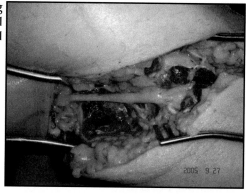

relieves tension on the nerve as is traverses the knee. We also recommend ensuring that the affected limb is not resting in a position that would contribute to external compression of the peroneal nerve, particularly at the level of the fibular head. Should an intrinsic cause, such as a postoperative hematoma, be identified and the neuropathy does not expeditiously resolve, then urgent surgical intervention is warranted. If an adequate decompression can be obtained, the hematoma should be aspirated without delay. Otherwise, formal hematoma evacuation should be performed with careful attention to hemostasis. Should the cause be related to an intraoperative procedure that may have caused partial or complete transection, such as pie-crusting for severe valgus/flexion contractures, then an early return to surgery for decompression, neurolysis, and potential nerve repair is appropriate.

The timing and need for surgical exploration and/or decompression of the nerve is controversial. We often see clinical improvement by three weeks. If there has been no clinical motor or sensory improvement by 6 weeks, we obtain electrodiagnostic studies consisting of electomyography (EMG) and nerve conduction studies (NCS) of the affected extremity. If these 6-week results demonstrate a neural regeneration pattern, then we serially observe our patients for continued improvement until recovery. However, if no improvement has been seen at 6 weeks or the patient has failed to demonstrate anticipated clinical recovery, then the clinical and electrodiagnostic studies are repeated at 3 months. Should the 3-month repeat studies fail to show neural regeneration and there is no improvement in clinical function, then surgical decompression is pursued.[2,7,8] Decompression entails a posterolateral longitudinal or diagonal incision centered at the head of the fibula. After opening the deep fascia, the nerve is most readily identified proximally at the biceps femoris tendon and followed distally until it enters the peroneus longus musculature (Figure 29-1). The nerve is fully released from all fibrous bands and the peroneus longus proximal attachment to the fibular head is released with any constricting septa. An intraneural neurolysis can also be performed at this point.

Further conservative measures include an ankle-foot orthosis for foot-drop and passive ankle range of motion exercises. Should the foot-drop persist, other options that have been described include tibialis posterior tendon transfers, tibialis anterior tenodesis, and peroneal nerve grafting.

The prognosis for recovery of a peroneal nerve palsy following total knee arthroplasty varies with the severity of initial symptoms and patient comorbidities. In our series, 68% of patients showed complete recovery by 18 months, which is consistent with other series.[1,3] In our experience, the majority of partial peroneal nerve palsies will fully recover while less than half of complete motor and sensory palsies recover without operative management. With intervention, the prognosis for recovery is nearly equal and the duration to maximal recovery is decreased. However, good functional capacity after TKA can be expected even with partial recovery.[3]

References

1. Schinsky MF, Macaulay W, Parks ML, et al. Nerve injury after primary total knee arthroplasty. *J Arthroplasty*. 2001;16:1048.
2. Mont MA, Dellon AL, Chen F, et al. The operative treatment of peroneal nerve palsy. *J Bone Joint Surg Am*. 1996;78(6):863.
3. Nercessian OA, Ugwonali OFC, Park S. Peroneal nerve palsy after total knee arthroplasty. *J Arthroplasty*. 2005;20:1068.
4. Idusuyi OB, Morrey BF. Peroneal nerve palsy after total knee arthroplasty: assessment of predisposing and prognostic factors. *J Bone Joint Surg*.1996;78A:177.
5. Knutson K, Leden I, Sturfelt G, et al. Nerve palsy after total knee arthroplasty in patients with rheumatoid arthritis. *Scand J Rheumatol*. 1983;12:201.
6. Horlocker TT, Cabanela ME, Wedel DJ. Does postoperative epidural analgesia increase the risk of peroneal nerve palsy after total knee arthroplasty? *Anesth Analg*. 1994;79:495.
7. Krackow KA, Maar DC, Mont MA, et al. Surgical decompression for peroneal nerve palsy after total knee arthroplasty. *Clin Orthop*. 1993;292:223.
8. Dellon AL. Postarthoplasty "palsy" and systemic neuropathy; a peripheral-nerve management algorithm. *Ann Plast Surg*. 2005;55:638.

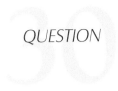

What Criteria Do You Use for a Manipulation Under Anesthesia?

Harpal Singh Khanuja, MD

The classic indication for manipulation after total knee arthroplasty (TKA) has been less than 90 degrees of flexion at 6 to 8 weeks postoperatively. While this remains an important guideline, a number of other factors should be taken into account.

When the patient presents in the acute postoperative period after a TKA with limited motion, it is imperative to review the history and the radiographs before considering intervention. Postoperative range of motion is closely related to preoperative motion.[1] Documenting the range of motion prior to surgery and at the time of wound closure, will help understand the progress or lack thereof in knee flexion. The hospital course should also be reviewed to determine if there were any postoperative complications that may have affected the range of motion. These could include a hematoma, or medical complications that may have led to a delay in rehabilitation.

Often the stiff postoperative knee is painful, and other causes for a painful knee such as infection need to be ruled out. This can be done clinically.

The radiographs need to be scrutinized for technical errors that may lead to the stiffness. Assessments include alignment, location of the joint line, and prosthetic size. Potential errors include "overstuffing" of the joint with too large a femoral component, or under-resection of the patella. These could lead to limited flexion. The joint line should be evaluated for patella baja.

If there does not appear to be a technical reason for the decreased motion, and you feel the patient is not close to the expected motion—based on preoperative and intraoperative ranges—a manipulation is warranted.

While 90 degrees of flexion at 6 weeks is a good guideline, it is not absolute. I typically decide at the 6-week postoperative visit if a patient will require manipulation. All patients are told preoperatively they are expected to have 90 degrees of flexion at 2 weeks, and if they do not obtain this by 6 weeks they will require manipulation. At the 6-week visit if they are close to 90 degrees, I stress the importance of improving motion over the next 1 to 2 weeks. If this does not improve they are told they will need to return to the operating room for a manipulation. It is important that this is communicated to the patient's therapist and family. The frequency of therapy visits may need to be increased for the unmotivated patient. Adequate pain control is also imperative during this period. The patient is assessed 2 weeks later, and if they have not made significant gains, a manipulation is scheduled. I like to perform manipulations in the first 8 weeks, although there is literature to support it can be beneficial up to 3 months.[2] If patients have less than 80 degrees at their 6-week visit, they will be scheduled for a manipulation.

The amount of flexion is not the only factor that is important to determine if a manipulation is necessary. How the patients progress postoperatively is just as important. If a patient had 30 degrees of flexion at discharge and is making little progress, it is reasonable to consider a manipulation sooner rather than later. Patients with poor flexion at discharge should be closely monitored for improvement.

Manipulations are routinely done on an outpatient basis. I use general anesthesia. Often muscle relaxation is not necessary. The hip is flexed. I place one hand on the joint line and my other hand at the level of the tibial tubercle—holding the leg lower creates a significant lever arm. Slow, gentle pressure is applied, and I feel and listen for the breaking of adhesions. You can lean with your chest and upper body on the proximal tibia to generate more force for larger legs. At the end of the procedure, range of motion is recorded and I will take a picture of the knee so the patient and family can witness the motion that was obtained. It is important that the postmanipulation therapy is coordinated. We arrange for the patient to have therapy that day, and again adequate pain control is important. I typically prescribe anti-inflammatories and oral narcotics for the postmanipulation period. The patient is discharged home to a formal therapy program at least 3 times a week. The patient is seen again at 2 weeks to make sure progress is made.

I do not routinely use CPM or epidurals after a manipulation and have not found the need to do so. This is supported by other studies.[3] I would consider this for a second manipulation, which is infrequent.

References

1. Lee DC. Intraoperative flexion against gravity as an indication of ultimate range of motion in individual cases after total *knee arthroplasty.* 1998;13(5).
2. Bong MR. Stiffness after total knee arthroplasty. *J Am Acad Orthop Surg.* 2004;12(3).
3. Keating EM. Manipulation after total knee arthroplasty. *J Bone Joint Surg Am.* 2007; 89(2).

I HAVE A PATIENT WHO FELL 3 MONTHS POSTOPERATIVELY AND FRACTURED THEIR PATELLA. SHOULD I TRY AND FIX IT?

Craig J. Della Valle, MD
Daniel J. Berry, MD

When faced with the patient who has a periprosthetic fracture of the patella, it is easiest to think about these fractures as belonging to one of three categories (Table 31-1). The available studies from multiple centers regarding the treatment of these injuries[1-5] demonstrate several clear trends. The first is that Type I fractures (those with a stable implant and an intact extensor mechanism) do very well with nonoperative treatment. The second is that operative treatment is associated with a very high rate of complications (>50%), reoperations, and failure to obtain union.

The high complication rate of operative treatment is probably due to a number of factors. First, the blood supply to the patellar remnant has previously been compromised by an arthrotomy and in some cases, a lateral release. Any fracture that is associated with poor blood supply has a high risk of nonunion. Second, it is difficult to gain fixation in the thin bone of the patellar remnant that is left if the patella has been resurfaced (periprosthetic fractures of the patella are rare in the unresurfaced patella). Finally, it is difficult to balance immobilization required for healing to occur against the stiffness that may result with extended immobilization.

About half of all periprosthetic patellar fractures are associated with an intact extensor mechanism and a well-fixed patellar component (Type I). Many Type I fractures are noted only as an incidental radiographic finding. For patients with an acute type I fracture a short course of immobilization followed by progressive protected range of motion in a hinged drop-lock knee brace typically will provide successful treatment.

Table 31-1

Classification of Periprosthetic Fractures of the Patella[4]

- Type I: Patellar implant is well fixed and the extensor mechanism is intact.
- Type II: Patellar implant is well fixed but the extensor mechanism is disrupted.
- Type III: Patellar implant is loose but the extensor mechanism is intact.

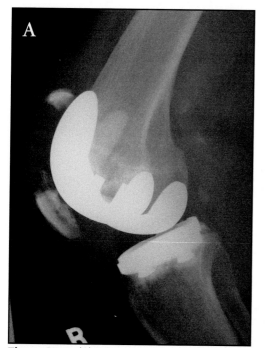 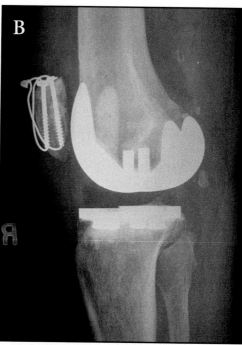

Figure 31-1. (A) A 78-year-old male presented after a fall with a displaced periprosthetic fracture of the patella and a disrupted extensor mechanism (Type II fracture) 18 months following primary total knee arthroplasty. (B) Three-month postoperative radiograph showing fixation with a tension-band and cannulated screws.

Over a quarter of periprosthetic patellar fractures are associated with a loose implant but an intact extensor mechanism (Type III fractures). Many of these are associated with osteonecrosis of the patella. Even if the patellar component is loose, if the patient can straight leg raise, initial treatment is nonoperative. If after several months time the loose patellar component becomes symptomatic, it can be removed or revised electively. When remaining bone stock is good, patellar revision may be considered, but in most cases the patella is thin or fragmented and the component is simply removed and the remaining patellar bone contoured to optimize tracking.

Because of the often poor results, operative treatment is only undertaken as an acute treatment for the fracture if the extensor mechanism is disrupted (a Type II fracture; Figure 31-1). If the extensor mechanism is not intact, the patient will not be able to ambulate unless continuity of the extensor mechanism is restored and unfortunately this requires operative treatment.

If operative treatment is required for a disrupted extensor mechanism, ensure that the skin overlying the anterior aspect of the knee is intact; if severe bruising or an abrasion is present, wait for the skin to heal. Expose the knee using a midline skin incision and clear the fracture site of hematoma. If adequate bone stock is present, the use of cannulated, partially threaded screws with a tension band wire running through the screws is biomechanically strongest.[2] Unfortunately, oftentimes there is inadequate bone stock present to accommodate cannulated screws and thus alternative methods such as a standard tension band or a circumferential cerclage must be employed. If the patella is osteonecrotic or the displaced fragment is small or otherwise difficult to fix, tendon advancement and extensor mechanism repair should be undertaken as opposed to attempted internal fixation. The surgeon must also understand that patellar fractures often are associated with femoral or tibial component malalignment or malrotation, and full revision total knee arthroplasty may be required in some cases.

If operative treatment is undertaken and fails, repeated internal fixation attempts are discouraged as the risk of infection is high and the chance of union low. In these circumstances, ongoing nonoperative measures may be considered. When a salvage operation is needed, an extensor mechanism allograft (see Question 46) may be considered.

Periprosthetic fractures of the patella are uncommon; however, treating them is a challenge. Patients who sustain this injury should be educated regarding the high rate of complications associated with operative treatment of this injury.

References

1. Berry DJ. Patellar fracture following total knee arthroplasty. *J Knee Surg*. 2003;16:236-241.
2. Carpenter JE, Kasman RA, Patel N, Lee ML, Goldstein SA. Biomechanical evaluation of current patella fracture fixation techniques. *J Orthop Trauma*. 1997;11:351-356.
3. Keating EM, Haas G, Meding JB. Patella fracture after total knee replacements. *Clin Orthop*. 2003;416:93-97.
4. Ortiguera CJ, Berry DJ. Patellar fracture after total knee arthroplasty. *J Bone Joint Surg Am*. 2002;84:532-540.
5. Parvizi J, Kim K, Oliashirazi A, Ong A, Sharkey PF. Periprosthetic patellar fractures. *Clin Orthop*. 2006;446:161-166.

I HAVE A PATIENT WHO TRIPPED AND FELL 3 MONTHS AFTER A TOTAL KNEE ARTHROPLASTY AND HAS A SUPRACONDYLAR FEMUR FRACTURE. WHAT IS THE OPTIMAL METHOD OF TREATMENT?

Mark Dumonski, MD
Walter Virkus, MD

We have found that the classification system developed by Lewis and Rorabeck is helpful in characterizing periprosthetic supracondylar total knee arthoplasty (TKA) fractures in that it addresses both fracture displacement and implant stability; the two main factors that affect our decisions in management.[1] Type I fractures are nondisplaced with a stable prosthesis; type II are displaced fractures with a stable prosthesis (Figure 32-1) and type III fractures denote a loose prosthesis.

Type I and II fractures can be treated nonoperatively, with open reduction and internal fixation (ORIF) or with retrograde intramedullary (IM) nailing. Nonoperative treatment requires prolonged immobilization and is associated with post-treatment stiffness and patient deconditioning and thus we reserve nonoperative treatment for patients who were nonambulatory prior to their fracture or who have severe medical comorbidities that make the risks of surgery prohibitive.

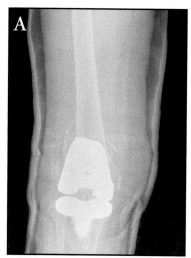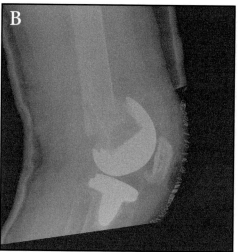

Figure 32-1. A type II supracondylar periprosthetic fracture in a 68-year-old woman with rheumatoid arthritis on chronic prednisone. The patient fell from a standing height. (A) Anterior-posterior view. (B) Lateral view.

Retrograde Intramedullary Nailing

Retrograde IM nailing is an attractive option in that surgical dissection at the fracture site is minimized and it is a biomechanically stable construct. The fracture, however, must be proximal enough to allow for at least two and preferably three distal locking screws. If retrograde nailing is chosen, proper preoperative planning is essential to identify whether or not the intercondylar notch of the femoral component is open (particularly in posterior stabilized total knee arthroplasties), if it is open how big the opening is (to determine whether or not the chosen nail will fit) and to arrange for both replacement and trial polyethylene spacers to allow for a modular polyethylene exchange at the time of surgery. The intercondylar distance of a TKA ranges from 12 to 22 mm, while standard retrograde nail diameters range from 9 to 15 mm.

It is important to recognize that the nail will not reduce the fracture in these distal metadiaphyseal fractures, and therefore we pay particular attention to both sagittal and coronal plane alignment throughout the reaming process, nail insertion, and distal locking. We find that it is particularly helpful to place a bump beneath the thigh to allow for flexion of the hip and knee that relaxes the deforming musculature. Care must be taken to avoid shortening the femur when comminution is present.

Locking Plates

Plate and screw constructs can also be used when treating a periprosthetic fracture and in general. We prefer to use locking compression condylar plates (Figure 32-2) as they allow the surgeon to use either standard or locked screws. Locked screws are desirable as they act as a fixed angle construct; this is particularly helpful in very distal fractures that involve small distal segments of osteopenic bone. Not only do locking plates increase

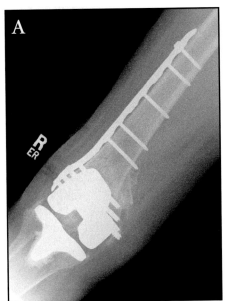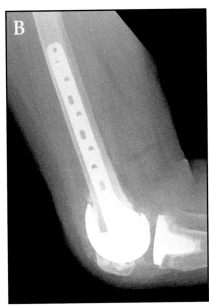

Figure 32-2. Postoperative radiographs following open reduction and internal fixation with a lateral locking compression plate. (A) AP view. (B) Lateral view.

biomechanical strength (when compared to plates that utilized nonlocking screws), their design facilitates percutaneous placement.[2] With a percutaneous technique, the soft tissue envelope and blood supply are largely maintained, thereby enhancing fracture healing. If an open technique is desired or required (because an adequate reduction cannot be obtained closed), soft-tissue stripping at the fracture site should be minimized.

Choosing Between a Retrograde Nail and a Locking Plate

If we are faced with a larger distal fragment (fracture begins above the flange of the femoral component and thus distal fixation can be achieved easily) and the make of model of the total knee components are known (so that the presence of an open box and its size is confirmed and replacement polyethylene liners are available) our first choice is a retrograde nail.[3] Once the patient is anesthetized, the ability to perform a closed reduction is confirmed and if an adequate reduction is obtained, we proceed with retrograde nailing. Locking plates are our preference in cases where the fracture is more distal as the current generation of locking plates allow for multiple points of distal fixation (often times 5 to 7 screws) even in very distal fractures such as those that start at the flange of the femoral component (see Figure 32-1B). They are also ideal if the presence of an open box cannot be confirmed, if replacement liners cannot be obtained, or if there is an ipsilateral total hip arthroplasty.

Component Revision

In type III fractures, the prosthesis is loose and must be revised. If bone stock is adequate, the failed component can be revised to a standard, revision stemmed component, bypassing the fracture site with a press-fit, canal filling, cementless stem and then achieving rotational stability with a plate and screws. If the bone stock of the distal femur is felt to be inadequate to support a standard revision femoral component, the distal femur can be replaced using either an allograft prosthetic composite (APC) or a distal femoral replacing modular oncology prosthesis. An APC is constructed by cementing a stemmed femoral component into a distal femoral allograft and then rigidly fixing the allograft to the remaining distal femur. Advantages of a distal femoral replacing modular oncology type prosthesis include relative ease of the surgical technique compared to an APC and the ability to immediately fully weight bear on the extremity if the femoral component is cemented. Further, no healing is required; however, if the construct fails secondary to loosening or infection, salvage can be difficult.

References

1. Lewis PL, Rorabeck CH: Periprosthetic fractures. In: Engh GA, Rorabeck CH, eds. *Revision Total Knee Arthroplasty.* Baltimore, MD: Williams & Wilkins; 1997:275-295.
2. Ricci WM, Bolhofner BR, Loftus T, Cox C, Mitchell S, Borrelli J. Indirect reduction and plate fixation with grafting, for periprosthetic femoral shaft fractures about a stable intramedullary implant. *JBJS Am.* 2005;87:2240-2245.
3. Gliatis J, Megas P, Panagiotopoulos E, Lambiris E. Midterm results of treatment with a retrograde nail for supracondylar periprosthetic fractures of the femur following total knee arthroplasty. *J Orthop Trauma.* 2005; 19:164-170.

How Do You Manage Acute Extensor Mechanism Disruptions?

Cory L. Calendine, MD
Kevin B. Fricka, MD

Disruption of the extensor mechanism following total knee arthroplasty is a potentially catastrophic complication. While many disruptions present late to our practice, acute management of these injuries is preferred.

The quadriceps tendon, patella, and patellar tendon provide three distinct regions of the extensor mechanism susceptible to failure. Establishing the exact location of the disruption by physical examination and radiographs guides our management. Most important, however, is evaluating the patient's level of disability. This information combined with a global understanding of the patient's health and expectations is vital to clinical success. Refer to Figure 33-1 for a graphic illustration of our treatment algorithm for extensor mechanism disruptions.

Bony disruptions of the extensor mechanism (patellar fractures) are treated somewhat differently than tendinous disruptions. If knee extension is maintained (regardless of fracture displacement), we treat these patients with short-term bracing and early weight bearing. If an extensor lag >10 degrees exist, we prefer surgical intervention for open reduction internal fixation versus partial patellectomy and tendo-osseous repair through bone tunnels versus patellectomy in extreme cases. We attempt to save the patellar component, if stable. It is important to understand, however, that operative treatment of these fractures is associated with high rates of complications and repeat procedures.

For a patient with a tendinous disruption of the extensor mechanism, we weigh the following treatment options: (a) observation with immobilizer, (b) direct primary repair, (c) direct primary repair with augmentation, and (d) reconstruction.

Nonoperative treatment is reserved for those who have minimal extensor lag (<10 degrees) or in whom a medical contraindication to surgery exists. In our hands, allowing these patients to be immediately full weight bearing in a knee immobilizer for 4 to 6 weeks has provided clinical success with minimal morbidity.

Figure 33-1. Treatment algorithm for extensor mechanism disruptions.

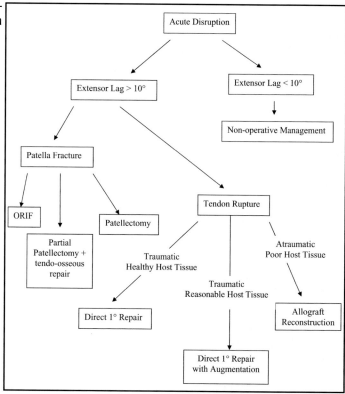

Direct primary repair can be performed using suture through bone tunnels, suture anchors, or tension band wiring; however, several authors have reported poor outcomes with direct repair. This is not unexpected because patients who suffer tendon disruptions often have weakened collagenous tissue secondary to systemic disease (inflammatory arthroplasties, diabetes, or renal failure) or steroid treatments (local injections or systemic). For this reason, we reserve primary repair for traumatic injuries in individuals with healthy host tissue. Our preferred technique for repair uses two #2 fiberwire sutures with a Krackow tendon stitch passed through three bony tunnels (the inner suture for both stitches is passed trough the middle tunnel) for tendo-osseous fixation.

Most patella or quadriceps tendon ruptures after total knee arthroplasty will require augmentation along with the primary repair. For proximal disruptions (quad tendon), a quad turndown is helpful. For distal disruptions, two techniques have been described. Cadambi and Engh[3] describe a technique in which the semitendinosus is left attached to the tibia distally and transected approximately 25 cm proximally through a separate posteromedial incision. The semitendinosus tendon is delivered through the midline incision, routed along the medial border of the patellar tendon, through the center third of the patella via a 5 mm drill hole, and sutured back to itself while holding the leg in extension. Postoperatively, these patients are immobilized in full extension for 8 weeks with partial weight bearing. When the integrity of the repair is confirmed at 8 weeks, motion is begun in a hinged range of motion brace starting at 0 to 30 degrees with 10 degree advancement per week.

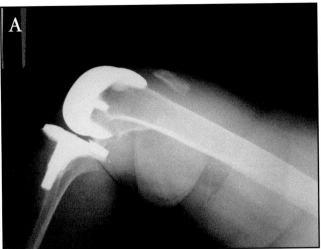

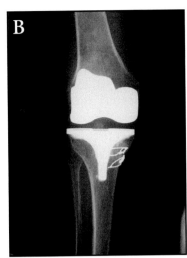

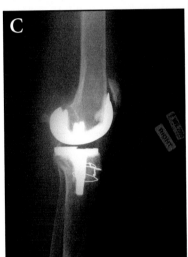

Figure 33-2. 67-year-old female with a history of Charcot-Marie-Tooth disease who underwent total knee arthroplasty with an unresurfaced patella. Two weeks postoperatively she sustained an acute patella tendon disruption. This was fixed with a tendo-osseous repair through drill holes and augmented with an Achilles tendon bone block allograft. She is able to ambulate with a cane and has a minimal extensor lag. (A) Lateral view demonstrating patella tendon rupture. (B and C) Postoperative AP and Lateral radiographs demonstrating repair technique with Achilles tendon augmentation.

Crossett and Rubash[2] describe another technique of augmentation with an Achilles tendon allograft. Primary repair is attempted and the Achilles tendon is used to augment the repair by securing the calcaneal bone block into a medial proximal tibia trough. This bone block is secured with a screw or cerclage wires (Figure 33-2). The Achilles allograft is then tensioned to the native tissue in full extension or hyperextension. The original technique describes draping the allograft over the repaired arthrotomy; however, we have tensioned it through the native quadriceps and repaired the arthrotomy over the allograft to maximize host tissue coverage of allograft tissue. The knee is not flexed after fixation and post-operatively rehabilitation is the same for semitendinosus augmentation.

Good outcomes in this devastating complication can be salvaged with these techniques. In our hands, we prefer the Achilles tendon allograft technique for augmentation of primary repairs. Crossett[2] and Cadambi[3] both demonstrated increased knee and functional scores after augmentation, improvement in range of motion, restoration of quadriceps strength (at least 4/5), and significant decrease in extensor lag with most being less then 5 to 10 degrees.

Unfortunately, frequently acute extensor mechanism disruptions occur in individuals with poor tissues leaving reconstruction as the best option. Reconstructions have been described using either allograft Achilles tendon bone block or the entire allograft extensor mechanism (quad tendon, patella, patellar tendon, and tibial tubercle). In these cases with poor host tissue and a disrupted extensor mechanism, we prefer reconstruction with the entire allograft extensor mechanism. Irrespective of your choice of allograft, we believe the best results occur when the allograft is fully tensioned in extension, native host tissue is sewn over the allograft, the allograft patella is not resurfaced, and the knee is immobilized in full extension with touch-down weight bearing for 8 weeks, after which a directed progressive physical therapy program is begun.

While acute disruptions of the extensor mechanism remain a challenging problem, careful assessment of the patient's health and disability combined with an understanding of all options will lead the surgeon to the ideal treatment for each patient.

References

1. Schoderbek RJ, Brown TE, Mulhall KJ, et al. Extensor mechanism disruption after total knee arthroplasty. *Clin Orthop.* 2006;446:176-185.
2. Crossett LS, Sinha RK, Sechriest VF, Rubash HE. Reconstruction of a ruptured patellar tendon with Achilles tendon allograft following total knee arthroplasty. *J Bone Joint Surg Am.* 2002;84-A:1354-1361.
3. Cadambi A, Engh G. Use of semitendon autogenous graft for rupture of the patellar ligament after total knee arthroplasty. *J Bone Joint Surg.* 1992;74A:974-979.
4. Burnett RS, Berger RA, Paprosky WG, Della Valle CJ, Jacobs JJ, Rosenberg AG. Extensor mechanism allograft reconstruction after total knee arthroplasty. A comparison of two techniques. *J Bone Joint Surg Am.* 2004;86-A:2694-2699.

SECTION IV

REVISION QUESTIONS

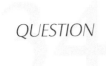
HOW DO YOU EVALUATE THE PATIENT WITH A PAINFUL TOTAL KNEE ARTHROPLASTY?

Michael J. Archibeck, MD

The cause of pain following total knee arthroplasty (TKA) can be determined in most cases with a thorough history, examination, the selective use of labs, and radiographic studies.

History

Typically my line of questioning includes the following topics: What is the primary complaint? Is it pain, stiffness, instability, or a combination of issues? Is there a prior history of infection or surgery on the knee? Were there any complications at the time of the index surgery (prolonged drainage, antibiotic use, an unusual amount of pain, a prolonged hospitalization, etc)? Was the preoperative knee pain relieved for a period of time? What is the character of the pain? Where is it located? When is it present—only with activity, at all times, at rest, with stairs? Does anything make it better? How far can you walk? Do you have to use a cane, crutches, or walker? Can you work?

Patients that are unhappy from the time of index surgery may have extrinsic sources of pain (back, hip, vascular), infection, complex regional pain syndrome, or gross surgical error. Patients that have good initial pain relief and subsequent pain often have mechanical sources of pain (loosening, wear) or late sepsis. Night or rest pain is often an indication of inflammation (infection, bursitis, tendonitis) or complex regional pain syndrome. Start up pain that improves slightly after a bit of walking and then worsens with further activity is suggestive of loosening. Symptoms of instability can be the result of ligamentous laxity, but I find more commonly are the result of quadriceps atrophy or patellar tracking issues.

Examination

Don't forget to examine potential extrinsic sources of pain (back, hip, vascular status). I generally group my exam into gait, sitting, and supine tests. Watch the patient's gait for an antalgic limp, alignment, instability, and the appearance of the foot (planovalgus, etc). Sitting exam with the legs dangling over the side of the bed includes inspection of rotation (in-toeing or out-toeing can indicate component rotational malalignment), a judgment about the girth of the quadriceps, an evaluation of flexion stability (coronal plane and assessment of posterior cruciate ligament [PCL] integrity in cruciate retaining [CR] TKAs), and an evaluation of patellar tracking with active flexion and extension against gravity or resistance. Supine exam includes a hip and spine exam (active and passive straight leg raise and hip range of motion [ROM]), palpation for effusion and tenderness (pes bursitis, tendonitis, neuromas, component overhang), an assessment of stability (coronal and sagittal plane), and an assessment of active and passive ROM of the knee (extensor lag).

Labs

I obtain a complete blood count (CBC), erythrocyte sedimentation rate (ESR), and C-reactive protein (CRP) in all painful TKAs. The CBC is rarely productive but the white blood cell count can be elevated in acute infection. The ESR and CPR (noncardiac) are essential in the assessment of possible infection.[1] I would also suggest that aspiration (off antibiotics) be performed routinely in the painful TKA (send for cell count with differential, crystal analysis (gout can occur in TKA), culture and sensitivity). If infection is suspected and the initial aspiration is not productive, the aspiration should be repeated to increase sensitivity. A synovial fluid white blood count of greater than approximately 2,500 cells/mm^3 and greater than 60% polymorphonuclear cells is highly suggestive of infection.[2] In the future, neutrophil gene expression may become a very effective test to identify infection.

Radiographic Studies

I routinely get a weight bearing anteroposterior view of both knees, a nonweight bearing lateral view, a merchant view, and a long standing radiograph of the entire extremity. Comparison to old radiographs is invaluable if available. These are inspected for signs of loosening (progressive radiolucencies, subsidence, cement mantle fracture), polyethylene wear and/or osteolysis, component sizing, overall limb alignment, and patellar tracking. If patellar tracking is abnormal, or if the patient's symptoms seem to be patellofemoral in origin, I obtain a CT scan to assess component rotational alignment.[3] I rarely find radionucleotide studies (technetium 99, indium 111 white blood count, sulfur colloid) to be helpful but occasionally obtain them in cases of diagnostic dilemma. If they are normal (which they rarely are) this essentially eliminates the possibility of loosening or chronic sepsis. Serial studies may demonstrate significant progressions or resolution. The reported sensitivity (64 to 100%), specificity (60 to 80%) of these studies, alone or in combination, is relatively poor.

Special Tests

I will occasionally use some form of injection as an aid to diagnosis. This may include an intra-articular injection of a local anesthetic to discern intrinsic from extrinsic sources of pain, a bursal injection (most commonly pes anserine), or injection of a suspected neuroma.

Common Causes of Pain Following TKA

Extrinsic Causes

* Hip
* Spine or radiculopathy
* Vascular claudication
* Complex regional pain syndrome

Intrinsic Causes

* Mechanical causes (related to TKA)
  * Loosening or failure of ingrowth
  * Instability (coronal or sagittal plane)
  * Polyethylene wear/ synovitis
  * Patellofemoral instability/pain
* Nonmechanical causes (tissues about the knee)
  * Infection
  * Inflammation
    * Bursitis
    * Tendonitis
    * Particulate synovitis
    * Neuroma

Conclusion

While the attached list of potential pain sources is not exhaustive, this categorization of the source can be useful and accounts for a great majority of cases. If, after the aforementioned evaluation, the etiology remains unknown I would tend to observe the patient at regular intervals (3 to 6 months) as early loosening or sepsis will eventually declare itself. I would strongly discourage "exploratory surgery" as this is rarely productive and can clearly worsen the patient's condition. If the diagnosis remains elusive, I will often send the patient for a second opinion.

References

1. Spangehl MJ, Masri BA, O'Connell JX, Duncan CP. Prospective analysis of preoperative and intraoperative investigations for the diagnosis of infection at the sites of two hundred and two revision total hip arthroplasties. *J Bone Joint Surg Am.* 1999;81(5):672-683.
2. Mason JB, Fehring TK, Odum SM, Griffin WL, Nussman DS. The value of white blood cell counts before revision total knee arthroplasty. *J Arthroplasty.* 2003; 18(8):1038-1043.
3. Berger RA, Rubash HE, Seel MJ, Thompson WH, Crossett LS. Determining the rotational alignment of the femoral component in total knee arthroplasty using the epicondylar axis. *Clin Orthop.* 1993;(286):40-47.

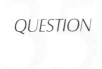

WHAT IS THE BEST TEST FOR DIAGNOSING PERIPROSTHETIC INFECTION?

Craig J. Della Valle, MD

When evaluating the patient with a painful total knee arthroplasty (TKA), infection must always be considered in the differential diagnosis, as treatment of the infected total knee is fundamentally different than the aseptically failed TKA. The diagnosis of infection is particularly difficult to make as there is no gold standard, multiple tests are available, and interpreting the tests that are available can be difficult. Although there are several good intraoperative tests for potentially identifying an infection, I prefer to make the diagnosis preoperatively so that I can better counsel the patient and prepare them for a two-stage exchange if an infection is identified.

The first tests that I order are an erythrocyte sedimentation rate (ESR) and c-reactive protein (CRP). In my own experience evaluating a consecutive series of 105 consecutive TKAs that underwent reoperation, the ESR and CRP (using a cut-off of 30 mm/hr and 10 mg/dl, respectively) were excellent screening tests, missing only one infected case.[1]

If either of these tests are abnormal, or if the history if very suggestive of infection (eg, history of diabetes, rheumatoid arthritis, prolonged antibiotic use around the time of the index arthroplasty, or wound healing problems) the knee is aspirated. The aspiration is performed using an 18-gauge needle and the fluid is sent for a cell count with differential and cultures including aerobic, anaerobic, fungal, and acid fast bacilli. It is important that the patient is off of antibiotics for at least 2 weeks prior to the aspiration or the cultures may be falsely negative.[2]

In my experience, the cell count is the best perioperative test for identifying infection. Using a cut-off of 3,000 wbc/ml, I found the synovial fluid white blood cell count to have a sensitivity of 100%, specificity of 98%, positive predictive value of 98%, negative predictive of 100%, and the accuracy to be 99%. Other authors have confirmed the value of perioperative cell counts in identifying the infected TKA, although Mason et al[3] recommended a cut-off of 2500 whereas Trampuz et al recommended a cut-off value of 1700.[4]

The cell count differential has also been recommended as a useful test for identifying infection with a differential of greater than 65%[3] or 80%[4] having been shown to be suggestive of infection although in my experience the cell count is a better test.[1]

There are instances where no fluid can be obtained in the office or where the patient declines an aspiration, and in these cases the surgeon must rely on intra-operative tests. My preference is to aspirate the knee in the operating room as a cell count can usually be performed in less than 40 minutes. The alternative is to send periprosthetic tissues (preferably synovial tissues adjacent to the implants) for an intraoperative frozen section. I use an average of ten polymorphonuclear cells in the five most cellular fields as my criteria for infection.[5] Polymorphonuclear cells are only counted if identified in tissue (and not fibrin) and if the surgeon is going to rely on frozen sections, a dedicated pathologist should be identified and the criteria used for infection should be agreed on so that intraoperative findings can be communicated effectively. Intra-operative gram stains are not an effective test and should not be relied on as a screening tool for infection as the sensitivity is poor.[7]

At the time of surgery, if the patient has not already had a negative pre-operative aspiration (cell count of less than 3000 wbc/ml and negative cultures) then three sets of operative cultures are obtained. Three sets of cultures are taken to help identify falsely positive results; one positive culture is more likely to be considered falsely positive if the overall clinical picture is one of aseptic failure whereas two cultures that are positive for the same organism are highly suggestive of infection. Cultures unfortunately can be both falsely positive and negative and if the picture is in any way unclear, an infectious disease consultation is obtained.

I rarely order nuclear medicine studies (such as indium labeled white blood cell scans), as they are expensive and only useful when negative; a negative result can reliably exclude infection while falsely positive results are common.[8] These tests are only ordered if the patient has a painful TKA and revision surgery is not otherwise indicated and the presence of infection cannot otherwise be ruled out (eg, the ESR and CRP are elevated, however no fluid was obtained at the time of aspiration).

In conclusion, I have found a peri-operative synovial fluid cell count to be the best test for identifying infection. This test is easily obtained, inexpensive, and can be performed either preoperatively or intraoperatively. Further, it is objective (as opposed to a frozen section) and its utility is supported by several studies in the literature.

References

1. Della Valle CJ, Sporer SM, Jacobs JJ, Berger RA, Rosenberg AG, Paprosky WG. Perioperative testing for sepsis in revision total knee arthroplasty. *J Arthroplasty.* 2007;22(6 suppl 2):90-93.
2. Barrack RL, Jennings RW, Wolfe MW, Bertot AJ. The Coventry Award. The value of preoperative aspiration before total knee revision. *Clin Orthop.* 1997;(345):8-16.
3. Mason JB, Fehring TK, Odum SM, Griffin WL, Nussman DS. The value of white blood cell counts before revision total knee arthroplasty. *J Arthroplasty.* 2003;18:1038-1043.
4. Trampuz A, Hanssen AD, Osmon DR, Mandrekar J, Steckelberg JM, Patel R. Synovial fluid leukocyte count and differential for the diagnosis of prosthetic knee infection. *Am J Med.* 2004;117:556-562.
5. Lonner JH, Densai P, DiCesare PE, Steiner G, Zuckerman JD. The reliability of intraoperative frozen sections for identifying active infection during revision hip or knee arthroplasty. *J Bone Joint Surg Am.* 1996;78:1553-1558.

6. Della Valle CJ, Bogner E, Desai P, et al. Analysis of frozen sections of intraoperative specimens obtained at the time of reoperation after hip or knee resection arthroplasty for the treatment of infection. *J Bone Joint Surg Am.* 1999;81:684-689.

7. Della Valle CJ, Scher DM, Kim YH, et al. The role of intraoperative gram stains in revision total joint arthroplasty. *J Arthroplasty.* 1999;14:500-504.

8. Joseph TN, Mujtaba M, Chen AL, et al. Efficacy of combined technetium-99 sulfur colloid/indium-111 leukocyte scans to detect infected total hip and knee arthroplasties. *J Arthroplasty.* 2001;16:753-758.

IF I AM DOING A REVISION TOTAL KNEE AND CAN'T SEEM TO GET ADEQUATE EXPOSURE, WHAT SHOULD I DO?

Craig J. Della Valle, MD

Gaining exposure at the time of revision total knee arthroplasty is an integral step in performing the procedure. The goals of this portion of the operation include protecting the skin, avoiding damage to the extensor mechanism, and providing visualization for both removing the existing implants and accurately preparing the bony surfaces for the revision implants. I achieve exposure by following a step-wise approach that gradually releases the extensor mechanism.

Once in the operating room, I incise the skin and create full thickness skin flaps as the blood supply to the skin comes from the deep fascia. If multiple skin incisions are present, I choose the most lateral one that will afford adequate access to the extensor mechanism as the blood supply to the skin of the anterior aspect of the knee is primarily derived medially. If the plane of dissection is unclear, I extend the incision beyond the old scar until normal tissue planes are identified. With the knee flexed, I make a medial parapatellar arthrotomy and perform a medial release. The medial release should be generous enough to allow the surgeon to externally rotate and deliver the tibia out of the wound and generally extends to the posteromedial corner of the tibia.

The next step is to re-establish the medial and lateral gutters. I start medially by identifying the junction between the medial joint capsule and the underlying scar with the knee extended (Figure 36-1). The interval between these planes can be developed using a knife or a sharp scissor. I then do the same laterally, developing a plane underneath the extensor mechanism between the quadriceps tendon and the underlying scar. The extensor mechanism is further released off of the femur proximally by passing a finger or an elevator underneath the quadriceps tendon.

Next, the interval between the patellar tendon and the tibia is developed using an electrocautery by placing a curved Homan retractor between the tendon and the tibia. I take great care at this point to avoid damaging the patellar tendon in any way and extend the

Figure 36-1. Identify the interval between the capsule and scar beneath it (blue line).

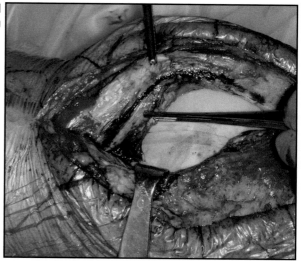

dissection around the tibia laterally as far as I can to allow excursion of the patellar tendon away from the tibia. Finally, the modular polyethylene liner is removed and my attention is turned toward the patella.

In general, I sublux the patella laterally and do not evert it as I find that eversion is unnecessary for wide exposure and places the patellar tendon at higher risk for avulsion. If I am having difficulty subluxing the patella laterally, scar and/or osteophytes can be removed from the lateral side of the patella and if subluxation is still a problem, a lateral retinacular release can be performed from inside out from the vastus lateralis proximally to the proximal tibia distally. In my experience the steps that I have described will provide adequate exposure for the majority of cases, even in stiff knees.[1]

If I cannot adequately expose the knee using the steps previously described, my first move is to perform a quadriceps snip.[2] A quadriceps snip is performed by extending the arthrotomy obliquely across the quadriceps tendon (proximally and laterally) at an angle of approximately 45 degrees (Figure 36-2). A snip is easily performed and the postoperative rehabilitation protocol need not be altered. Both clinical studies and my own experience have shown that these patients have no differences in strength, clinical scores, or range of motion when compared to those who have not required a snip for exposure.[3,4]

If exposure is still suboptimal (which is uncommon), the extensor mechanism can either be fully released proximally with a V-Y quadricepsplasty (later modified by Insall and called the patellar turndown[5]) or released distally with a tibial tubercle osteotomy[6] (TTO). A V-Y turndown is performed by extending the arthrotomy distally along the lateral border of the extensor mechanism. Potential benefits of this approach include the ability to lengthen the extensor mechanism although this often leads to an extensor lag. A TTO is preferable in my experience and offers the advantage of greater access to the tibial canal; in my mind a TTO is most useful as an adjunct to removing fully cemented revision stems from the tibia or in cases of extreme patella baja. To perform a TTO, extend the skin incision distally and use a saw to make a coronal cut from the most proximal portion of the tibial tubercle distally for 6 to 8 cm maintaining a bone bridge at the proximal extent to resist proximal migration of the fragment once repaired. The osteotomy is levered open

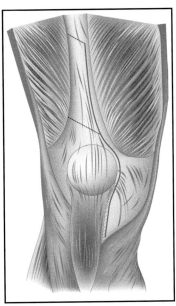

Figure 36-2. Schematic representation of a quadriceps snip. The proximal, dark dotted line represents the preferred level for crossing the quadriceps tendon; the more distal, lightly dotted line is not recommended secondary to a higher risk of extensor mechanism rupture. (Adapted from Nelson CL, Kim J, Lotke PA. Stiffness after total knee arthroplasty. *J Bone Joint Surg.* 2005;87:264-270.)

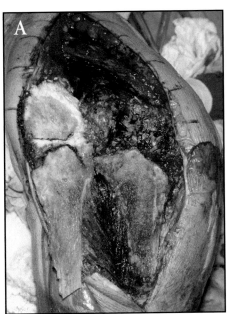

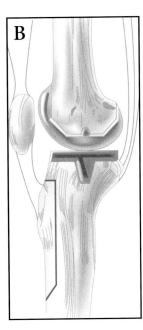

Figure 36-3. (A) Clinical photograph of the exposure afforded by a tibial tubercle osteotomy; note the severe contracture of the patellar tendon. (B) Schematic representation of the bony cuts used for a tibial tubercle osteotomy. (Adapted from Nelson CL, Kim J, Lotke PA. Stiffness after total knee arthroplasty. *J Bone Joint Surg.* 2005;87:264-270.)

with wide osteotomes maintaining the soft-tissue sleeve laterally. The knee is then gently flexed and the patella everts. Closure of the osteotomy is performed with three 16 gauge wires that are looped between drill holes made in the lateral aspect of the tubercle fragment and the medial aspect of the proximal tibia.

References

1. Della Valle CJ, Berger RA, Rosenberg AG. Surgical exposures in revision total knee arthroplasty. *Clin Orthop.* 2006;446:59-68.
2. Garvin KL, Scuderi G, Insall JN. Evolution of the quadriceps snip. *Clin Orthop Relat Res.* 1995;321:131-137.
3. Barrack RL, Smith P, Munn B, et al. The Ranawat Award. Comparison of surgical approaches in total knee arthroplasty. *Clin Orthop Relat Res.* 1998;356:16-21.
4. Meek RM, Greidanus NV, McGraw RW, Masri BA. The extensile rectus snip exposure in revision of total knee arthroplasty. *J Bone Joint Surg Br.* 2003;85(8):1120-1122.
5. Aglietti P, Windsor RE, Buzzi R, Insall JN. Arthroplasty for the stiff or ankylosed knee. *J Arthroplasty.* 1989; 4(1):1-5.
6. Whiteside LA. Exposure in difficult total knee arthroplasty using tibial tubercle osteotomy. *Clin Orthop Relat Res.* 1995;(321):32-35.

WHEN DOING A REVISION TOTAL KNEE, DO YOU START RECONSTRUCTING THE FEMUR OR TIBIA FIRST?

David G. Nazarian, MD

Revision knee arthroplasty requires the surgeon to restore a mechanically sound arthroplasty in a previously failed joint. Of course, an understanding of the specific modes of failure germane to the particular knee are necessary criteria to achieve a successful reconstruction. Adequate exposure to the knee allows the surgeon to better understand the problems of the prior reconstruction and avoid them in the nascent arthroplasty.

Once the knee is fully exposed, it is my preference to extract and reconstruct the tibial component first. It is important to visualize the entire surface of the failed tibial implant by fully releasing the deep fibers of the medial collateral ligament and semimembranosus and excision of the entire infrapatellar fat pad. Full eversion of the patella greatly enhances both tibial and femoral exposure. The patellar tendon insertion may be protected with a towel clip placed through a burr hole (Figure 37-1). The femoral implant left in place allows you to use this as a buttress in order to lever and dislocate the tibia anteriorly with a sharp Homan retractor. This retractor will also protect the neurovascular structures posteriorly.

I prefer to use a small-blade oscillating saw to disrupt the bond between the implant and cement or bone. Curved osteotomes are used to circumferentially disrupt the entire proximal tibial connection (Figure 37-2). A straight impaction tool now may be used to extract this component. If a tibial stem extension is currently well-fixed in place then the tibial surface component should be disconnected in order to gain access and remove the well-fixed stem with mechanical or ultrasonic tools. The tibial surface may be freshened with a 0 degree cutting guide. I choose a system with a non sloped component in order to make rotational adjustments at any time during the arthroplasty. The canal is reamed to achieve a tightly press-fit stem. My preference is to use a 75 mm cementless stem extension unless a diaphyseal defect necessitates a longer stem or a capacious canal would be better served with cement fixation. An offset stem may be used to help translate the tibial component more laterally to improve patellar tracking.

Figure 37-1. Full eversion of patella and protection of tendon insertion with towel clip.

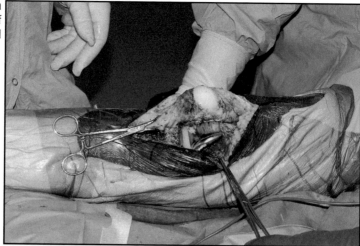

Figure 37-2. Disruption of tibial component achieved with 1/2″ curved osteotome.

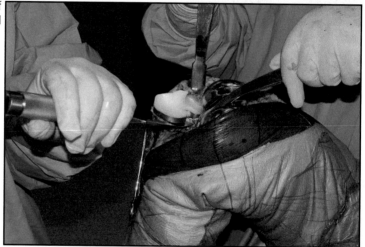

The tibial reconstruction serves as a stable foundation on which to perform the remainder of the arthroplasty. Tibial rotation may be assessed by the position of the tibial tubercle (Figure 37-3). Because the tibia symmetrically affects the flexion and extension gaps, it is easier to perform this part of the arthroplasty first. I use hemitibial augments when there is a medial or lateral defect larger than 5 mm or a complete augment when the joint line cannot be restored or the flexion and extension gaps cannot be filled with the thickest polyethylene tibial insert. Block or wedge augments can be fit to the tibial tray undersurface and into the area of deficiency. I will choose a tibial size that achieves maximum bone contact with minimal overhang.

The more complex portion of the arthroplasty involves appropriate sizing and positioning of the femoral component. A general rule of thumb is to reconstruct the distal and posterior femur with the size implant and augments that restore the joint line to either 2.5 cm below the femoral epicondyles, 1 cm above the fibular head, or at the level of the meniscal scar. The distal femur affects the extension gap while the posterior femur affects the flexion gap. The interplay

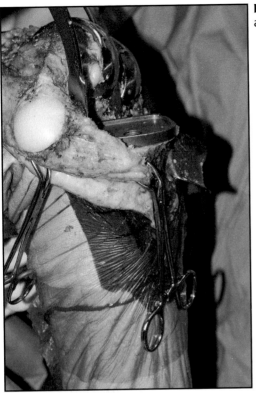

Figure 37-3. Assessment of tibial trial position and rotation.

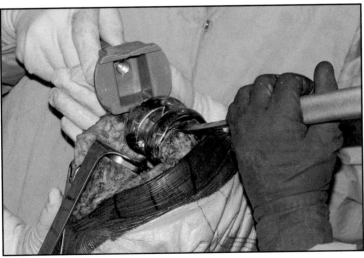

Figure 37-4. Removal of femoral component with osteotomes.

between implant size and the use of augments will help appropriately position the femoral component in space in order to achieve flexion/extension gap matching.

I removed the femoral implant with 0.5-inch and 0.25-inch curved osteotomes inserted at the prosthetic/cement interface or prosthetic/bone interface in cementless implants (Figure 37-4). Usually the component can be rendered loose and disimpacted without causing significant bone damage. I have found the use of power tools to be an

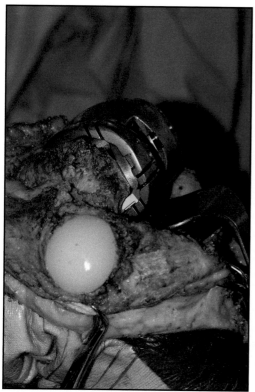

Figure 37-5. Femoral trial component in position with augments.

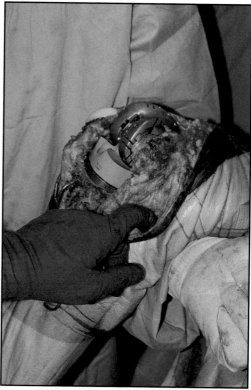

Figure 37-6. Femoral liftoff used to test collateral ligament competence in flexion.

unrewarding exercise during femoral implant removal, but it is helpful in removing residual cement adherent to the femoral bone. The use of distal femoral augments will help restore the joint line, which is often raised in revision surgery. I generally choose a size implant that allows anterior/posterior prosthetic contact with the host bone. A posterior lateral augment will help ensure appropriate external rotation (Figure 37-5). If a flexion gap is significantly larger than the extension gap then a larger femoral implant with posterior augments will decrease the size of the flexion gap. I recommend choosing a 75 mm or 135 mm stem depending on the quality of the metaphyseal bone. An offset stem may afford more appropriate femoral positioning for a patient's particular anatomic requirements. Once the trial tibial and femoral components are firmly in place I choose the thickness of tibial polyethylene spacer that restricts femoral liftoff and flexion, but allows full extension (Figure 37-6). In addition, when the knee is placed in full extension, if the tibia is appropriately externally rotated then lining up the center of the components will further ensure proper femoral rotation (Figure 37-7). I always begin trialing with a posterior stabilized insert to better estimate collateral ligament competence and determine the amount of constraint required.

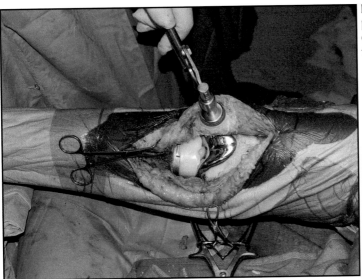

Figure 37-7. Center of components aligned in extension ensures symmetric tibial and femoral rotation.

Assessment of the patella begins with inspection of the retained implant. If it is minimally worn, well positioned, and is less than 25 mm in thickness then I recommend leaving the patellar component in place. Final range of motion and patellar tracking observation are the concluding trial steps before cementing the chosen implants.

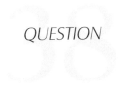

SHOULD I USE STEMS ON ALL OF MY REVISION TOTAL KNEE COMPONENTS?

Steven H. Weeden, MD
Wayne Paprosky, MD

Revision total knee components are commonly stemmed to protect the limited autogenous bone stock that remains. Revision components utilized in primary total knee arthoplasty (TKA) without stems may place higher than normal stresses upon the often compromised bone particularly if a more constrained articulation is required to obtain stability. If bulk allograft or trabecular metal augments are anticipated, a stem must be used to protect the reconstruction. With joint loads being several times body weight, a stemmed component can transfer loads to the normal and more robust bone of the diaphysis. There are few conditions that the authors would not utilize a stem during revision TKA.

A stem's purpose is to transmit force away from the joint line; once a stem reaches 70 mm in length, the axial load at the joint line can be reduced by 23% to 39%. Conversely, stems up to 15 cm in length may result in stress shielding of the proximal tibial cortex and doubling of the strain located at the tip is noted. A shorter stem is typically used on the tibia (where end of stem pain is more of a concern) and longer stems are used on the femur. The option of cementing or press-fit technique is discussed in another section. It is essential that the revision surgeon realize that stems are an adjunct to obtaining stability and not a substitute for obtaining optimal metaphyseal coverage of the revision component.

Presently, most cementless stems are smooth or blasted without a porous coating. Flutes have been added to the stems to aid in fixation and decrease stiffness. Flutes or splines on the stem engage in endosteal bone and function to decrease rotational stresses. Flutes may also act to decrease the modulus of elasticity of the stems and thus decrease proximal stress shielding and end of stem pain.

Preoperative Planning

Full-length anteorposterior and lateral radiographs allow for assessment of the femur and tibia. In addition to determining the position of the joint line, alignment of bony cuts, size and placement of components and need for augmentation, the intramedullary canals are assessed to ensure that intramedullary alignment will restore accurate mechanical axis orientation. It is useful to template for at least two stem lengths and their corresponding stem diameters. For structural bulk allografts, stem fixation along the endosteal bone should have cortical contact and should occur two or more canal diameters past the graft into the diaphyseal bone.

Operative Technique

Preparation of the femoral and tibial bony surfaces is done using intramedullary alignment guides. Rather than using narrow intramedullary guide rods, the authors promote the use of intramedullary reamers (or trial rods) for the cutting-jig. The initial step is to ream and push the largest diameter reamer past the isthmus until endosteal cortical contact is felt or heard. Cutting blocks are then attached to this rod and initial cuts are completed. By using the largest diameter rod in the canal and ensuring that the rod passes the isthmus, one can better assure that the bony cuts for the component will correlate to the stem orientation and prevent impingement or malpositioning of the component-stem construct.

It is essential to reiterate that the position of the femoral and tibial components is dictated by the position of the stem if the stem is canal filling. If the canal is eccentric or the tibial plateaus deficient, then a base plate with an offset housing or offset stem will need to be considered to optimize coverage of the tibial plateau. The authors use an offset stem in approximately 60% of tibial revisions (Figure 1). With the femoral component, an offset stem can be used to adjust the flexion gap, optimize patellar tracking by lateralizing the component or prevent impingement of the femoral component against the anterior cortex of the femur. The authors use an offset stem in approximately 40% of femoral revisions.

Traditionally, we ream approximately 1 cm past the tip of the stem to ensure that there is no tip impingement or cortical erosion. For routine revisions, reaming should not be overly aggressive. Stem insertion and reaming proceeds line to line. Final components are then inserted in a routine manner. If components are cemented at the joint (which is recommended), cement should extend to the stem-component junction.

Conclusion

In conclusion, successful revision total knee arthroplasty routinely includes stemmed components for long-term survival and joint function. Offset stems on the tibia are useful to optimize proximal tibial coverage and femoral offset stems can assist with gap balance, patellar tracking and alignment.

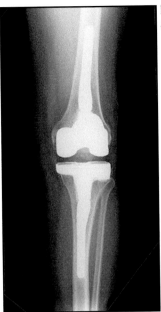

Figure 38-1. An offset tibial stem is used during revision TKA to assist with proximal bone-implant coverage.

Bibliography

Weeden SH, Paprosky WG. *Use of Stems in Revision Total Knee Arthroplasty. The Adult Knee.* Lippincott, Williams & Wilkins; 2003:1439-1446.

Bertin KC, Freeman MAR, Samuelson KM, Ratcliffe SS, Todd RC. Stemmed revision arthroplasty for aseptic loosening of total knee. *J Bone Joint Surg (BR)* 1985;67:242-248.

Haas SB, Insall JN, Montgomery W, Windsor R. Revision total knee arthroplasty with use of modular components with stems inserted without cement. *J Bone Joint Surg (AM).* 1995;77:1700-1777.

Paprosky WG. Use of distal femoral allografts in revision total knee arthroplasty. *Current Concepts in Primary And Revision Total Knee Arthroplasty.* Lippincott-Raven; 1996:217-226.

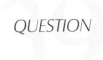

IF I USE A STEM AT THE TIME OF A REVISION TOTAL KNEE ARTHROPLASTY, SHOULD I PRESS-FIT THE STEM OR CEMENT IT?

Craig J. Della Valle, MD
Aaron G. Rosenberg, MD

Stems are widely used in revision total knee arthroplasty (TKA) to provide additional support for component fixation. They act to augment implant stability by off-loading deficient bone, and distribute fixations stresses in the face of the increased articular constraint often required in this and other clinical settings (see question 38). While widely accepted, it is unclear whether the stem should be fully cemented into place, or if a hybrid technique (where the metaphyseal region of the stem is cemented and the end of the stem is tightly fit into the diaphyseal bone; Figures 39-1 and 39-2) is optimal. Biomechanically, a short, cemented stem and a longer press-fit stem have similar properties in terms of augmenting strength of fixation[1,2] and thus to a certain extent the choice is a matter of surgeon preference, although specific attributes of one technique may be preferable in a specific clinical scenario.

Cemented stems have shown good intermediate term results and have a longer track-record.[3,4] Advantages of a fully cemented stem include immediate fixation, a relatively straight-forward surgical technique, and the ability to deliver local antibiotics (via antibiotic loaded cemented). In addition, the position of the component is not as constrained by the position of the stem and equivalent fixation may be achieved with less invasion of the intramedullary canal. However, cemented stems are usually more difficult to remove and have a greater potential for stress shielding of the off-loaded metaphyseal bone. Difficulty if removal is required is the most compelling reason to not utilize this technique routinely.

Advocates for using a canal-filling press-fit stem that is cemented only in the metaphysis site good short- to intermediate-term results[5,6] and the aforementioned equivalence

Figure 39-1. Revision TKA with a hybrid cementing technique where the metaphyseal portion of the stem is cemented and the remaining portion is tightly fit into the diaphysis. Our preference is to use cement just past the modular junction where the stem connects to the revision component. Note the use of an offset stem on the tibia that translates the component anteriorly and laterally.

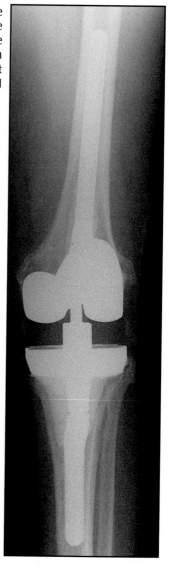

when tested biomechanically. The use of a canal filling, longer stem that engages the diaphysis has been associated with better component alignment[7] and is among the reasons why this technique is widely used. On the tibial side, if the stem engages the canal, prosthetic alignment will be neutral (or very close to neutral) and similarly, on the femoral, side the valgus alignment will be dictated by the fixed valgus angle present between the femoral component and the attached stem; alignment in the lateral plane is similarly assisted with a canal-engaging stem. End of stem pain has been described with the use of tightly fitting, diaphyseal engaging stems but seems to occur in only a small number of patients, typically resolves within 2 years of surgery and has been associated with solid, cobalt chrome stems whereas most modern systems today utilize titanium stems where this problem is seen less frequently.

What is clear, is that if a press-fit stem is utilized, it should engage diaphyseal bone and be tightly press fit into the canal and the concept of a so-called "dangling stem" does not provide

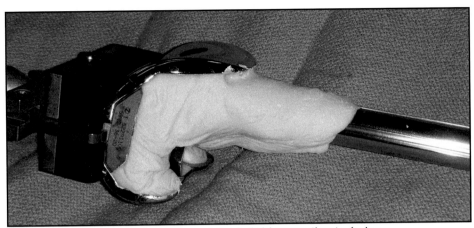

Figure 39-2. Intraoperative picture of the hybrid cementing technique.

adequate support and has been associated with a higher rate of failure.[3] The technique that we utilize includes a stem that is cemented proximally and press-fit distally in the majority of patients (see Figure 39-1). The surgical technique we use is described in Question 37.

Another potential disadvantage of a press-fit, canal-fitting long stem is that the stem to a certain extent will dictate the position of the tibial tray or the femoral component on the cut metaphyseal surface. This can potentially lead to undersizing the revision component so that it does not overhang the surface of the bone leading to suboptimal component size (which can lead to problems matching the femur and tibia in some systems and resultant instability) and decreased strength of fixation if the component is not contacting the intact cortical rim. Further, if the femoral or tibial component is not appropriately lateralized, patellar maltracking can result (see Question 13). This can be particularly problematic on the tibial side as the tibial canal is offset posteromedially with respect to the tibial plateau in many patients.

To solve this conflict, an offset stem is used in many tibial reconstructions and is required in some femoral reconstructions (see Question 40; Figure 39-1). Most manufacturers currently offer offset revision stems and this problem can usually be solved; however, in some cases where there is deformity of the canal, a short cemented stem is preferable. The other situation that oftentimes requires a shorter, fully cemented stem is when a hinged prosthesis is utilized. These components typically include a longer, nonmodular keel segment (75 mm in the system that we use) that houses the hinged mechanism and post. In this situation, it may be impossible to add on a press-fit stem extension and given the additional requirements for stability given their constrained nature, we usually fully cement the tibial tray when using a hinged revision component (Figure 39-3).

An additional consideration is the use of longer press-fit stems in shorter (predominantly female patients). Given their short stature, a stem of greater than 150 mm in combined length could potentially complicate treatment of a future proximal femoral fracture or hip arthritis if a prosthetic hip stem is required and in these patients I prefer to use a shorter press-fit or cemented stem. Finally, there are those patients in whom bone stock, even of the diaphysis, is poor and an acceptable press-fit cannot be obtained. If good stability cannot be obtained with the trial components, we will fully cement the stem to ensure adequate prosthetic stability.

Figure 39-3. A fully cemented tibial stem in a hinged revision TKA. The longer (75 mm) nonmodular keel of the tibial tray precludes the use of an additional stem extension in most patients. The femoral stem has been inserted using a hybrid technique with cement near the articular surface and a press-fit in the canal.

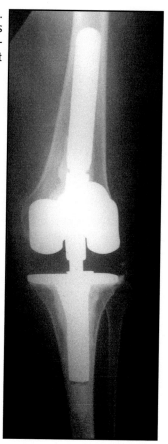

References

1. Jazrawi LM, Bai B, Kummer FJ, Hiebert R, Stuchi SA. The effect of stem modularity and mode of fixation on tibial component stability in revision total knee arthroplasty. *J Arthroplasty.* 2001;16:759-767.
2. Peters CL, Craig MA, Mohr RA, Bachus KN. Tibial component fixation with cement: full versus surface-cementation techniques. *Clin Orthop Relat Res.* 2003;409:156-168.
3. Fehring TK, Odum S, Olekson C, Griffin WL, Mason JB, McCoy TH. Stem fixation in revision total knee arthroplasty: a comparative analysis. *Clin Orthop Relat Res.* 2003;416:217-224.
4. Murray PB, Rand JA, Hanssen AD. Cemented long-stem revision total knee arthroplasty. *Clin Orthop Relat Res.* 1994;309:116-112.
5. Peters CL, Erickson J, Kloepper RG, Mohr RA. Revision total knee arthroplasty with modular components inserted with metaphyseal cement and stems without cement. *J Arthroplasty.* 2005;20:302-302.
6. Gofton WT, Tsigaras H, Butler RA, Patterson JJ, Barrack FL, Rorabeck CH. Revision total knee arthroplasty: fixation with modular stems. *Clin Orthop Relat Res.* 2002;404:158-168.
7. Parsley BS, Sugano N, Bertolusso R, Conditt MA. Mechanical alignment of tibial stems in revision total knee arthroplasty. *J Arthroplasty.* 2003;18:33-36.

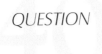
WHEN DO YOU USE AN OFFSET STEM DURING REVISION TOTAL KNEE REPLACEMENT?

Scott M. Sporer, MD, MS

Tibial and femoral stem extensions can be utilized to improve component fixation by allowing stress transfer to the intact bone of the more proximal femur and more distal tibia.[1-3] I utilize tibial and femoral stem extensions in all of my revision total knee arthroplasties as I believe this minimizes the chance of early failure as opposed to the use of primary components used in the revision setting. Although stems can be fully cemented into place, I prefer to use canal filling press-fit stems as in our group's experience they are associated with a low rate of failure and I find that they improve the patient's overall coronal and sagittal plane alignment. When using a canal filling stem, the stem will, to a certain extent, dictate the position of the tibial and femoral component; if a shorter or non-canal filling cemented stem is used, this does not occur as this type of stem will allow some degree of component translation.

In order to address this issue, offset stems are available that allow for 4 to 6 mm of anterior-posterior or medial-lateral translation (Figure 40-1). In addition to allowing the surgeon to optimize component coverage, these stems also allow the surgeon to fine-tune both patellar tracking and soft tissue balancing.[4]

I prepare the tibial surface first as the level of the tibial cut will affect both the flexion and extension gaps. The optimal joint line height can be determined based on the position of the fibular head (typically 10 mm proximal to this point) and a decision can be made regarding the need for tibial augments. I then use straight reamers inserted by hand (not on power) to size the diameter of the tibial canal and recut the proximal tibia using the reamer as an intramedullary cutting guide. I cut the tibia with no slope as the revision tibial component I prefer has seven degrees of slope built into it. Subsequently, I assess the location of the reamer within the tibial canal (in relation to the cut upper end of the tibia) to get an initial idea of where my stem will need to be to optimize tibial coverage. In general, the center of the medullary canal is situated in a posterior and medial position

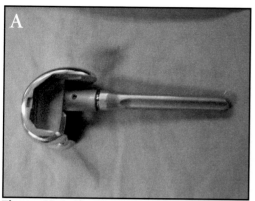 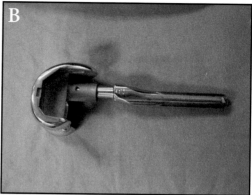

Figure 40-1. The stem extension can consist of either a (A) straight or a (B) offset extension of varying lengths. These stem extensions can provide additional component stability while maximizing host prosthesis–bone contact, improving soft tissue balancing, or improving patellar tracking.

Figure 40-2. Offset tibial stem extensions are frequently used in revision knee surgery to improve coverage of the tibial plateau. The offset extension is commonly used to shift the tibial tray anterior and lateral relative to the anatomic axis of the tibia.

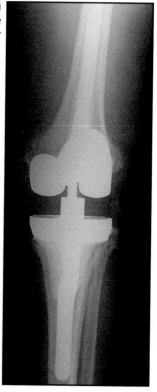

relative to the center of the tibial plateau and thus I usually need an offset stem that places the tibial component in a relative anterior and lateral position as compared to the canal (Figure 40-2). If a straight stem is chosen in this situation, the surgeon must either compromise the coverage of the tibial plateau and use a smaller component or risk a component that overhangs medially and/or posteriorly.

I now turn my attention to the femur. Most patients will require the use of distal femoral augments to restore the joint line and a posterior lateral augment to ensure an

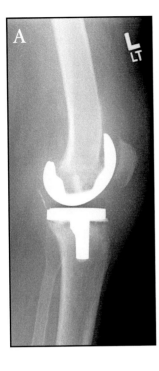
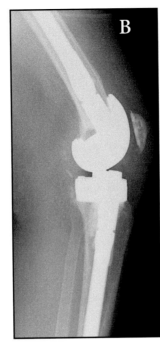

Figure 40-3. Offset femoral stem extensions are frequently used to preferentially adjust the flexion space by moving the femoral component in the anterior/posterior plane or to improve patellar tracking by moving the femoral component more lateral. (A) Preoperative radiographs of a patient with an aseptically loose femoral component. (B) Postoperative radiographs demonstrating a femoral stem shifting the femoral component posteriorly relative to the anatomic axis to improve flexion stability.

appropriate amount of femoral component external rotation to optimize patellar tracking. I initially perform a trial reduction of the femoral component with a long straight femoral stem extension. Most implant systems have a predetermined amount of valgus built into their components and this will verify that the coronal alignment is appropriate. A trial reduction can be performed assuming that the joint line has been appropriately recreated. I now assess the flexion and extension gaps noting any laxity or asymmetry between them. If both the flexion and extension gaps are loose, a larger polyethylene liner trial is inserted to "fill up" both gaps. However, this can lead to joint line elevation and if the patella is close to articulating with the polyethylene trial in deep knee flexion, I increase the amount of distal femoral augmentation to lower the joint line. This, however, can cause a flexion extension mismatch (too tight in extension but loose in flexion). In this situation, I will switch the straight femoral stem to an offset one to translate the femoral component posteriorly, which will preferentially "tighten up" the flexion space (Figure 40-3).

A similar situation can be encountered when a knee is stable in extension but is tight in flexion. In this scenario the femoral component can be preferentially translated anteriorly with an offset stem to "loosen up" the flexion space. However, if the femoral component is translated anteriorly, care must be taken to avoid overstuffing the patellar femoral joint, which can result in anterior knee pain and/or decreased knee flexion and if this is a concern, the alternative option is to downsize the femoral component if it fits the anatomy appropriately.

The medial-lateral position of the femoral component on the distal femur and patellar tracking are now assessed. An offset stem can translate the femoral component medially or laterally (to improve coverage of the femoral component) or the femoral component can be translated laterally to improve patellar tracking. I find that I need to use an offset stem on the femoral side much less frequently than I do on the tibia.

I believe that tibial and femoral stem extensions should be considered during most revision total knee arthroplasties. The use of an offset stem is an option in the surgeon's armamentarium to maximize implant coverage, preferentially adjust the flexion and extension gaps, and optimize patellar tracking.

References

1. Conditt MA, Parsley BS, Alexander JW, Doherty SD, Noble PC. The optimal strategy for stable tibial fixation in revision total knee arthroplasty. *J Arthroplasty*. 204;19(7 Suppl 2):113-118.
2. Langlais F, Belot N, Ropars M, Lambotte JC, Thomazeau H. The long-term results of press-fit cemented stems in total knee prostheses. *J Bone Joint Surg Br*. 2006;88(8):1022-1026.
3. Parsley BS, Sugano N, Bertolusso R, Conditt MA. Mechanical alignment of tibial stems in revision total knee arthroplasty. *J Arthroplasty*. 2003;18(7 Suppl 1):33-36.
4. van Loon CJ, Kyriazopoulos A, Verdonschot N, de Waal Malefijt MC, Huiskes R, Buma P. The role of femoral stem extension in total knee arthroplasty. *Clin Orthop Relat Res*. 2000;(378):282-289.

How Do You Handle Massive Bone Loss at the Time of Revision Total Knee Arthroplasty?

Allan E. Gross, MD, FRCSC, O.Ont
Oleg Safir, MD, FRCSC
David Backstein, MD, MEd, FRCSC

When considering the management of significant bone loss at the time of revision total knee arthroplasty, the classification which I use divides bone defects into contained, which means that there is an intact peripheral rim of bone, and uncontained.[1] If the defect is uncontained (segmental) it is either noncircumferential or circumferential. If it is non-circumferential only one condyle or one plateau is involved, whereas if it is circumferential, it affects both condyles or both tibial plateaus.[2]

The methods of reconstruction for loss of bone include excess cement plus or minus screws, autograft, metal augments, allograft, and tumor prostheses. All these techniques have their own indications. Parameters that must be considered are contained versus uncontained, size of the defect, location of the defect, and patient factors such as age, underlying medical conditions, and the capacity to heal and rehabilitate.[1,2] Contained and uncontained defects require stemmed components, and I use stems that are press-fit into the diaphysis with cement around just the proximal part of the stem that is within metaphyseal bone. For the elderly low demand patient with a small contained defect, I think that it is appropriate to use excess cement, which can be reinforced with screws, particularly on the tibial side. Screws are left protruding into the contained defect, and if they have a good solid purchase they reinforce the cement that is used to fill the contained defect. For larger contained defects morsellized bone graft should be impacted into the defect. The bone graft is usually a mixture of autograft that is found in the area and allograft. The bone graft has to be impacted firm enough so that a layer of cement between your implant and the bone graft is sitting on the surface of the impacted bone rather than going through it.

Uncontained defects should be managed by augments if they are within the dimension that can be addressed by the augments of the system that you are using. The size of augments that are available varies somewhat from system to system, but generally speaking are around 10 to 15 mm in thickness. On the femoral side augments can be applied distally, posteriorly, and some systems offer anterior augments. On the tibial side, augments can be applied as blocks or wedges on either the medial or lateral sides. You should also keep in mind that on the tibial side you can make up for much more substantial bone loss if it is circumferential because you can increase the thickness of your polyethylene up to 3 cm. It is important, however, that you not make up for femoral bone loss on the tibial side because that will raise the level of your joint line. To establish the level of the joint line, you can use either the lower pole of the patella or the top of the fibular head. Both are approximately one finger's width from the joint line.

When dealing with uncontained defects that are beyond the scope of augments, then you have to make a decision as to whether or not you are going to use a tumor prosthesis or a structural allograft. Tumor prostheses offer a shorter healing time and a faster rehabilitation. They are technically easier to do and there are no bone-to-bone interfaces that require healing. Stress fractures and resorption are not a problem. There are no donor problems, no storage problems, and they are not as adversely affected by chemotherapy or radiation. Tumor prostheses have the disadvantages of poor soft tissue and bone attachment, which is particularly relevant on the tibial side where the patellar tendon and tubercle have to be reattached. Violation of the host canal by cement or a porous coat is necessary. Revision is difficult because of failure to restore bone stock. A hinge is necessary, and in young patients, long-term implant loosening and stress shielding is going to make future revision very difficult.

Structural allografts have the advantages of soft tissue attachment, bone attachment, extensor mechanism attachment, no violation of host canal using our technique, which does not use cement or a porous coat in the canal. Re-revision is facilitated by restoration of bone stock, and available healthy host canal. Structural allografts have certain disadvantages such as longer healing time (union of the allograft bone to host bone interfaces can take time), the potential for nonunion, disease transmission, and the technically demanding nature of the procedure. It is very important for you to consider the patient profile when deliberating between a tumor prosthesis or a structural allograft. In my practice, tumor patients receive tumor implants and most revision patients receive structural allografts. Patients with malignancies benefit from a short rehabilitation, and also may have received chemotherapy and/or radiation, which inhibits the healing response of host bone to allograft. There is also a higher incidence of infection, and allograft bone provides a better nidus for bacterial contamination than tumor implants. The indications for structural allografts are any uncontained defect that is beyond the scope of implant augments in patients who you are unwilling to make the leap to a tumor prosthesis. Also, structural defects involving the patellar tendon insertion are dealt with by structural allografts to which tendon and bone can be reattached. Further, patients that are likely to require further surgery are probably better managed with structural allograft.

Structural allograft is used as an allograft implant composite for circumferential defects, or as a condyle or plateau when the defect is not circumferential. It is my opinion that deep frozen rather than freeze dried bone is preferable because it is at least 10 to 15% stronger. Noncircumferential grafts are fixed with 4.5 or 6.5 mm cancellous screws and protected by press-fit diaphyseal filling stems. The graft has to be fixed before instrumentation takes place. The implant surface is cemented to the graft, but the interface between graft and host has to be kept clear of cement in order for it to heal.[2]

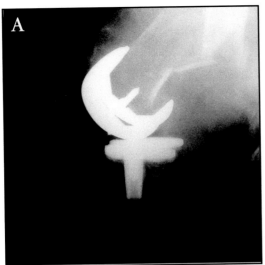 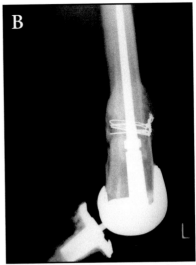

Figure 41-1. (A) Lateral x-ray supracondylar fracture 1 year after TKR. (B) Osteoporosis and comminution made internal fixation impossible so a distal femoral allograft composite implant was used to construct the knee.

The allograft prosthetic composite is used for circumferential defects beyond the scope of implant augments. The technique that we use for allograft implant composite reconstructions is to cement the graft to the implant except at the graft host junction and to use a press-fit diaphyseal filling stem. The junction between the host bone and the allograft should be either a step-cut or a long oblique cut in order to provide stability and enhance the probability of union. The stem beyond the allograft is not porous coated and not cemented. The allograft implant composite is prepared on a side table with trial reductions prior to cementation of the implant into the graft. Once a good fit is obtained with regards to joint stability, level of joint line etc, then cementation takes place on a side table. The graft is then inserted and the junction stabilized using 16-gauge cerclage wire. In addition, all of the residual host bone is wrapped around the allograft, particularly at the junction in order to provide more stability and also to enhance union. It is important to keep the soft tissues attached to this residual host bone because it contains capsule and the collateral ligaments that provide stability for the reconstruction. If the graft host junction is not absolutely solid, then you should apply a cortical strut allograft once again using cerclage wires as a biological plate to provide stability. I always use constrained components when doing an allograft prosthetic composite graft, using the maximum cam post mechanism in order to accomplish this. I do not use a rotating hinge. The identical technique is done on both the tibial and femoral sides, but our use of this technique is much more common on the femoral side because you can make up much larger defects on the tibial side because of the thickness of the polyethylene[2] (Figures 41-1 to 41-3).

We have published our results using this technique in the revision situation and our most recent data is as follows. We have performed 68 structural allografts in 61 knees with a clinical and radiographic follow-up of 5.5 years. Nineteen were done for periprosthetic fractures, 29 for loosening, 11 as part of a two-stage reconstruction for infection, and 2 for instability. Thirteen of 61 knees with 68 structural allografts failed due to graft-related complications. There was 1 nonunion, 3 aseptic loosening, 3 periprosthetic fractures, 4 infections, and 2 failures secondary to instability.[3,4]

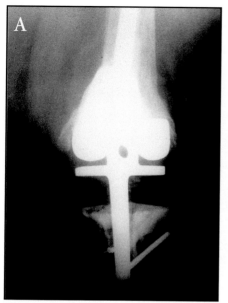
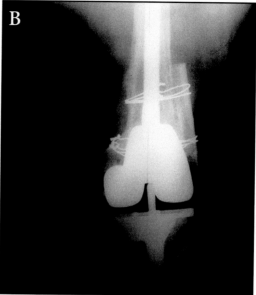

Figure 41-2. (A) AP x-ray of a TKR performed with thick poly to make up for distal femoral loss of bone stock. (B) Revision carried out with distal femoral structural allograft restoring the joint line to the correct level. A cortical strut allograft was used to help stabilize the graft host junction.

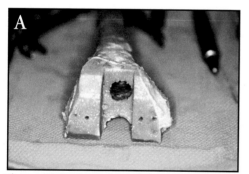
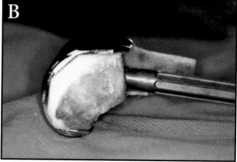

Figure 41-3. Circumferential graft technique. Distal femoral allograft has been instrumented (A) and then cemented to implant on a side table (B).

References

1. Ghazavi M, Stockley I, Gilbert Y, Davis A, Gross AE. Reconstruction of massive bone defects with allograft in revision total knee arthoplasty. *J Bone Joint Surg.* 1997; 79A(1):17-25.
2. Clatworthy MG, Balance J, Brick GW, Chandler HP, Gross AE. The use of structural allograft for uncontained defects in revision total knee arthoplasty: a minimum five-year review. *J Bone Joint Surg.* 2001;83A(3):404-411.
3. Kassab M, Zalzal P, Azores GMS, Pressman A, Liberman B, Gross AE. Management of periprosthetic femoral fractures after total knee arthroplasty using a distal femoral allograft. *J Arthroplasty.* 2004;19(3):361-368.
4. Backstein D, Safir O, Gross AE. Management of bone loss: structural grafts in revision total knee arthroplasty. *Clin Orthop Relat Res.* 2006;(446):104-112.

How Do I Decide if I Should Retain the Patellar Component at the Time of Revision Total Knee Arthroplasty?

Thomas E. Brown, MD
Khaled Saleh, MD, MSc, FRCSC
Quan Jun Cui, MD, MS
William Mihalko, MD, PhD

The fate of the patellar component during revision total knee arthoplasty (TKA) should be based on multiple factors: fixation of the component, status of the polyethylene, and the congruity of the old patellar component with the new femoral revision component. Following successful revision of the femoral and tibial components and reestablishment of a well balanced TKA, we turn our attention to the patella. First and foremost, we make certain that the patella tracks truly throughout a full range of motion. If maltracking exists, we reassess femoral and tibial component rotation to make certain that both components are appropriately rotated in the transverse plane. Correct rotation of the femoral and tibial components should be obtained before proceeding with a lateral retinacular release and/or medial reefing of the extensor mechanism. Unnecessary lateral release only further compromises the vascularity of the patella.

Once extensor mechanism balance is achieved, we assess the patellar component for signs of stability and wear. Prior to assessment, the patellar meniscus should be completely excised to assess tracking as well as the bone–cement interface. Any signs of cement cracking at the periphery or movement of the patellar component with respect to the bone should raise your suspicion for loosening. We also measure the thickness of the patellar construct to calculate the relative thickness of the remaining patellar bone, in the event revision is necessary. We closely inspect the surface of the patellar component to look for signs of severe damage or delamination. The relative congruity of the patellar component with the trochlea of the new femoral component should also be assessed. With a well-fixed and well-preserved patellar component that tracks centrally in the new trochlea, we will accept some incongruity in this new patellofemoral articulation.[1] The amount of polyethylene debris generated is small, and this eliminates the very real possibility of creating a patellar fracture intra-operatively during the removal of the patellar component, or revising the new component onto inadequate (<12 mm), potentially dysvascular patellar bone stock. If the composite thickness of the patella and component is >25 mm in females, or >28 mm in males, and the reason for TKA revision is knee stiffness or arthrofibrosis, we will revise the patella to decrease the composite thickness and hopefully improve flexion.

In the event that patellar component revision is needed, remove the old component with a wide, thin-blade oscillating saw, amputating the component at the base of the pegs. If the patella is metal backed, use a high speed metal cutting wheel to achieve the same result. You should avoid the temptation to pry the component off, as this frequently results in a patellar crack or fracture. Once the component is removed, you can remove the retained pegs and remaining cement with a burr and curettes. Remeasure the thickness of the remaining bone stock to determine how much, if any, additional bone you can remove.

Free-hand saw cuts of the remaining patellar bone are normally required, as the various patellar cutting jigs and reaming systems are difficult to position and stabilize on deficient bone stock. Be conservative with your cuts, shaving away bone, then remeasuring, and do not resect to below the depth of the existing peg holes unless the patella is excessively thick (>17 mm).

If you are faced with a situation in which the remaining patellar articular surface is concave, do not attempt to resect until you obtain a flat surface. This will likely result in a patellar fracture now or later. It is better to utilize a biconvex patellar implant that will fill this void and improve the composite strength of this construct (Genesis Biconvex Patella, Smith & Nephew, Memphis, TN, and TM patella, Zimmer Inc, Warsaw, IN).[2] If this shell of bone is excessively thin, it may be more prudent to either create a purse-string pouch and restore patellar thickness with impaction bone grafting,[3] or to leave the patella unresurfaced to avoid iatrogenic fracture. This so-called patelloplasty may result in some anterior knee pain, but this is certainly preferable to patellar fracture, component dissociation, and potential loss of extensor function.[4]

When cementing the patella to the remaining bone, carefully prepare the boney surface with a burr to create some interdigitation points for the cement. Be careful with creating additional peg holes—it may be safer to utilize one or more of the existing holes to avoid creating more stress-risers in this fragile bone. While compressing the prosthesis to the bone during cement polymerization, be careful not to exert too much force with the patellar clamp, as this can result in fracture even at this last stage.

In summary, retention of a well fixed, well preserved patellar component that tracks well in the trochlea is preferable to revision to minimize the risk of fracture and/or extensor mechanism disruption. If revision is required, careful removal, bone preparation, and appropriate implant selection should result in a successful patellar reconstruction.

References

1. Lonner JH, Mont MA, Sharkey PF, Siliski JM, Rajadhyasha AD, Lotke PA. Fate of the unrevised all-polyethylene patellar component in revision total knee arthroplasty. *J Bone Joint Surg Am.* 2003;85:56-59.
2. Maheshwer CB, Mitchell E, Kraay M, Goldberg VM. Revision of the patella with deficient bone using a biconvex component. *Clin Orthop Relat Res.* 2005;440:126-130.
3. Hanssen AD. Bone grafting for severe patellar bone loss during revision knee arthroplasty. *J Bone Joint Surg Am.* 2001;83:171.
4. Parvizi J, Seel MJ, Hanssen AD, Berry DJ, Morrey BF. Patellar component resection arthroplasty for the severely compromised patella. *Clin Orthop Relat Res.* 2002;397:356- 361.

How Do You Manage the Patient With Severe Patellar Bone Loss at the Time of Revision Total Knee Arthroplasty?

Kevin J. Bozic, MD, MBA
Michael D. Ries, MD

Patellar bone loss during revision total knee arthroplasty (TKA) may result from wear-induced osteolysis, patellar component loosening, fracture, infection, or implant removal. Severe patellar bone loss may compromise the integrity of the extensor mechanism. Our goals when treating the patella with severe bone loss in revision TKA are to maintain the integrity of the extensor mechanism, achieve central tracking of the patella, and provide mechanical support for a patellar component if possible to minimize anterior knee pain. Our decision making depends on the amount and quality of remaining bone stock, the fixation of the existing patellar component, and the integrity of the extensor mechanism.

Patellar bone loss in revision TKA can be treated with cemented biconvex patellar component revision, cementless trabecular metal patellar reconstruction, morcelized allograft, whole patellar allograft, patellectomy, or patelloplasty. In cases where the existing patellar component is not damaged and remains well fixed to host bone, we leave the patella component in place, even when there is a mismatch between the patella design and the trochlear groove of the patellar component given the high risk of potential problems if the component is revised.

The most important factor we consider when choosing among treatment options is the amount of remaining patellar bone stock. We have previously reported that the use of a cementless trabecular metal patellar component is associated with good results when at least 50% of host patella is remaining, but using this technique in the face of significant patellar bone loss (greater than 70%) results in a high rate of failure.[1]

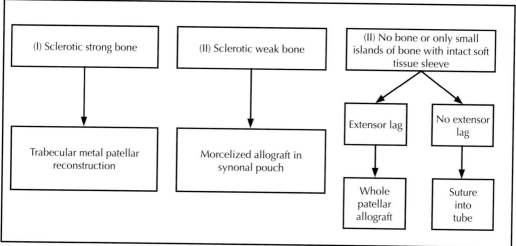

Figure 43-1. Classification of remaining patellar bone stock and algorithm for management of severe patellar bone loss.

We think about the remaining bone stock as separable into three basic categories: (1) sclerotic strong bone, (2) sclerotic weak bone (eggshell), and (3) no bone or only small islands of bone fragments with an intact soft tissue sleeve (Figure 43-1).

Cement penetrates well into cancellous bone and is most appropriate for patellar revision with minimal bone loss and preservation of the cancellous bone structure.[2] However, severe patellar bone loss is often associated with a sclerotic bony shell. Cement fixation into a sclerotic bone surface can result in early loosening. Removal of the previous patellar component with either debridement of prominent bone along the patellar rim (patelloplasty) or gull wing osteotomy to improve the shape of the patella and tracking in the trochlear groove avoid problems of revision resurfacing.[3,4] However, patelloplasty is often associated with anterior knee pain.[3] Cementless trabecular metal fixation has been associated with successful early results and offers a viable option to cemented patellar revision. We use this technique when the patella is sclerotic and cannot accommodate cemented fixation.[1] However, the remaining patellar bone stock should have adequate mechanical integrity to support the extensor mechanism. Implantation of a trabecular metal patella requires reaming to fit the component, which results in some additional bone loss and decrease in strength of the remaining patella. If the patellar bone stock is sclerotic and has poor mechanical integrity (eggshell), fracture may occur if the bone is reamed. In this situation, we have employed morcelized bone grafting to improve the strength of the patella and minimize risk of post-operative fracture. The morcelized bone is placed into a synovial pouch to contain the bone fragments until revascularization occurs.[5]

For management of complete patellar bone loss (prior patellectomy) or when only small islands of bone are present such as with severe osteolysis, but the extensor mechanism soft tissue sleeve is intact, trabecular metal patellar reconstruction can result in a high rate of loosening and necrosis of the extensor mechanism.[1] Whole patellar allografting with suture fixation of the allograft tendons to the extensor mechanism restores patellar height and improves extensor mechanism strength.[6] However, allograft resorption or infection may occur. We use this technique for patients with prior patellectomy and an extensor lag in whom quadriceps strength requires improvement and justifies the risk of allograft complications. If there is no extensor lag, then we suture the extensor mechanism soft tissue sleeve into a tube to allow it to track better in the femoral component trochlear groove rather than implant a solid bone graft.

References

1. Ries MD, Cabalo A, Bozic K, Anderson M. Porous tantalum patellar augmentation. The importance of residual patellar bone stock. *Clin Orthop.* 2006;452:166-170.
2. Graham J, Ries M, Pruitt L. Effect of bone porosity on mechanical integrity of the bone cement-interface. *J Bone Joint Surg.* 2003;85A:1901-1908.
3. Barrack RL, Matzkin E, Ingraham R, Engh G, Rorabeck C. Revision knee arthroplasty with patellar replacement versus bony shell. *Clin Orthop.* 1998;356:139-143.
4. Vince KC, Blackburn DC, Ortaaslan SG, et al. "Gull Wing" osteotomy of the patella in total knee arthroplasty. *J Arthroplasty.* 2000;15:254.
5. Hanssen AD. Bone-grafting for severe patellar bone loss during revision knee arthroplasty. *J Bone Joint Surg Am.* 2001;83:171-176.
6. Busfield BT, Ries MD. Whole patellar allograft for total knee arthroplasty after previous patellectomy. *Clin Orthop.* 2006;450:145-149.

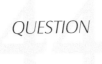

HOW DO YOU ASSESS JOINT LINE POSITION AT THE TIME OF REVISION TOTAL KNEE ARTHROPLASTY? WHAT ARE THE CLINICAL CONSEQUENCES IF IT IS ELEVATED?

Richard S. Laskin MD

Joint line malposition has been shown to lead not only to instability but also to an increased incidence of anterior knee pain and decreased flexion secondary to patellar infera and posterior soft tissue impingement by the femoral component. Thus, it is important to reposition the femoral component in its proximal-distal position at the time of revision total knee arthroplasty (TKA).

There are several landmarks that have been described to help determine the correct position of the joint line.

Landmark #1: **The tip of the fibular styloid** (Figure 44-1). The normal joint line lies approximately 10 mm proximal to the tip of the fibular styloid. There are only occasional patients in whom this landmark may not be accurate including those who have had a prior medial closing wedge osteotomy with proximal fibular resection and those with a history of severe tibial and fibular fracture. Because it is applicable in almost all cases, this is my preferred landmark.

Landmark #2: **The sulcus of the medial epicondyle** (Figure 44-2). The normal joint line lies approximately 25 mm distal to the sulcus of the medial epicondyle. Unfortunately the sulcus is often obscured by the overlying attachment of the medial collateral ligament, making its position difficult to properly ascertain.

Landmark #3: **The inferior pole of the patella**. The normal joint line lies approximately 5 mm distal to the inferior pole of the patella. Whereas this is a good landmark to use in the primary knee, patellar tendon shortening that often occurs after a knee replacement usually makes this landmark inaccurate in the revision situation.

Figure 44-1. The joint line typically lies 10 mm proximal to the tip of the fibular styloid.

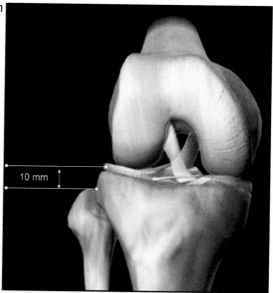

Figure 44-2. The joint line typically lies 25 mm distal to the sulcus of the medial epicondyle.

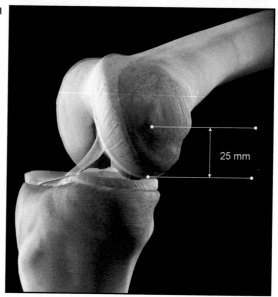

Landmark #4: **The position of the previous femoral component**. If the femoral component had been placed in the proper position at the time of the index knee replacement, its position can be used as a guide during the revision. Prior to its removal a caliper is used to measure a fixed distance proximal from the end of the prosthetic condyle. This point is marked on the anterior cortex of the femur with a cautery. After insertion of the revision trial prosthesis, its position is adjusted so that this distance is reproduced. The surgeon must recognize, however, that the original component may have been malpositioned proximally and in our experience this occurs in up to half of TKAs that require revision, particularly for instability.[1]

Using these landmarks, I normally proceed in the following manner:

1. I remove the femoral and tibial components. The tibial canal is then reamed until a snug fit is obtained.

2. A cutting block with an attached trial tibial stem the diameter of the last reamer used is seated and a freshening cut is performed.

3. A trial tibial base plate with the attached trial tibial stem is seated on the cut surface.

4. The femoral canal is reamed until a snug fit is obtained.

5. A cutting block of approximately the same size as the femoral component removed is affixed to the trial stem and seated so that the anterior cutting slot is aligned with the anterior surface of the femur. On occasion this may require the use of an offset adaptor on the stem. The anterior, posterior, and chamfer surfaces are then resected and a freshening cut of the distal femur is performed.

6. A trial femoral component of approximately the same anterior-posterior diameter as the femoral component that had been removed is affixed to a trial intramedullary stem and seated on the femur.

7. A tibial trial polyethylene is chosen so that the distance from its surface to the tip of the fibular styloid will be 1 cm.

8. The knee is checked for stability first in flexion. If the knee is loose in flexion, a large femoral component is inserted. The resultant space between the posterior surface of the bone and the inner posterior surface of the implant can be filled with augments.

9. If the extension space is too large it usually means that the femoral component was seated too far proximally and trial augments are used to move the component caudad until stability in extension is achieved.

The commonest mistake made by the "occasional" revision knee surgeon is to seat the femoral component on whatever remaining bone there is on the femur. This usually results in proximal displacement of the implant and the concomitant use of a revision femoral component that is too small; a thick polyethylene is then used to obtain stability in flexion and extension. Martin and Whiteside,[2] in a cadaveric study, demonstrated that proximal displacement of the joint line as little as 5 mm resulted in mid flexion instability. At full extension and at 90 degrees of flexion, the knees appeared stable; however, there was marked laxity in both the varus-valgus and rotatory planes at 30, 45, and 60 degrees of flexion. Similar findings have been reported by Sidles et al[3] in a computer generated model. Furthermore, as the joint line is elevated, patella baja results with impingement of the patellar implant on the front of the tibial component and resultant anterior knee pain and decreased flexion.[4]

In summary, the algorithm that we have described allows proper placement of the joint line as well as proper balancing of the flexion and extension spaces during revision TKA; two of the most important steps in performing a successful revision TKA.

References

1. Laskin, R. Joint line position in revision knee arthroplasty. *Clin Orthop.* 2002;404:169-171.
2. Martin JW, Whiteside LA. The influence of joint line position on knee stability after condylar knee arthroplasty. *Clin Orthop.* 1990;259:146-156.
3. Sidles JA, Matsen FA, Garlini JL, et al. Total knee arthroplasty: functional effects of tibial resection level. *Trans Orthop Res Soc.* 1986;12:263.
4. Figgie HE, Goldberg VM, Heipel KG, Miller HS, Gordon NH. The influence of tibial patellofemoral location on function of the knee in patients with the posterior stabilized knee prosthesis. *J Bone Joint Surg.* 1986;68A:1035-1040.
5. Yoshii, I, Whiteside LA, White SE, Milliano MT. Influence of prosthetic joint line position on knee kinematics and patellar position. *J Arthroplasty.* 1991;6:169-177.

WHEN SHOULD I USE A CONSTRAINED CONDYLAR INSERT AS OPPOSED TO A POSTERIOR STABILIZED INSERT?

Kelly G. Vince, MD, FRCS

"Constraint" in total knee arthroplasty designates a "mechanical substitution for deficient or removed ligaments." Accordingly, a posterior stabilized (PS) polyethylene articular insert uses a femoral cam and tibial post to reproduce some of the resistance to posterior tibial dislocation in flexion normally provided by the posterior cruciate ligament. By contrast, a constrained condylar (CC) insert has a taller tibial spine that conforms to a larger femoral intercondylar box and restricts varus-valgus and sometimes, rotation between the tibia and the femur. Most primary TKAs and approximately 40% of revisions can be stabilized with the size and position of posterior stabilized implants combined with soft tissue releases. Less constrained implants are generally favored, to decrease load on the fixation and maximize longevity of the arthroplasty.

The most common need for constraint in a primary arthroplasty is structural failure of the medial collateral ligament in a valgus deformity. Less commonly, severe varus deformity (usually with a pronounced thrust on ambulation) with structural failure (plastic deformation) of the lateral structures to the point where medial releases cannot balance the knee and may produce instability.

The two indications for constraint in revision surgery are: (1) instability in flexion despite implantation of the largest femoral component possible (fits medial to lateral) and a thick PS insert and (2) instability in extension secondary to collateral ligament failure.[1] Implant systems that can be easily converted from PS to CC minimize instrumentation and maximize efficiency in surgery. The conversion from PS to CC usually involves deepening the femoral intercondylar box and enhancing fixation with stem extensions.

Diagnosis of the cause of failure is essential prior to revision TKA (Table 45-1). A number of causes can account for instability, but only true ligamentous failure usually requires a constrained prosthesis (Figure 45-1). I find that computerized tomography (CT) is invaluable to determine component orientation that could lead to stiffness, exten-

Table 45-1

Causes of TKA Failure

1. Infection
2. Extensor mechanism rupture
3. Stiffness
4. Tibio-femoral instability
5. Fracture
6. Loosening
7. Patella complications and malrotation
8. Implant failure

Figure 45-1. Causes of instablility in TKA.

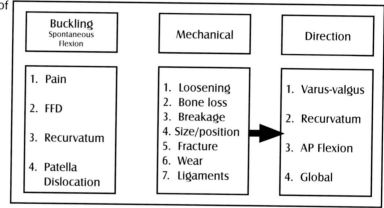

Buckling Spontaneous Flexion	Mechanical	Direction
1. Pain	1. Loosening	1. Varus-valgus
2. FFD	2. Bone loss	
	3. Breakage	2. Recurvatum
3. Recurvatum	4. Size/position	
	5. Fracture	3. AP Flexion
	6. Wear	
4. Patella Dislocation	7. Ligaments	4. Global

sor mechanism dysfunction, and instability.[2] Single leg AP and lateral weight bearing radiographs demonstrate dynamic instability in addition to loosening, component breakage, periprosthetic fracture, and sizing of the components. A 3-foot standing radiograph depicts mechanical limb alignment, which is critical in the evaluation of instability. This shows extra-articular deformities plus hip and ankle pathology that can contribute to instability.

I feel the choice between a PS and CC insert emerges logically from a systematic approach to revision arthroplasty, which differs from primary surgery. In virtually all cases, both femoral and tibial components should be revised; incomplete revisions are often unsatisfactory.[3] Among other problems of partial revisions, the option of constraint will usually not be available unless both components are changed. I favor, in general, intrameduallary fixation with stems long enough to engage the diaphyseal endosteum for superior fixation and control of alignment. Preoperative planning should signal the need for structural allograft bone, metal augments, porous metal augments, allograft ligaments, or allograft extensor mechanisms. Reconstitution of lost bone may be all that is necessary to restore functional tension to ligaments and provide stability without constraint.

A systematic three-step approach indicates when to select a CC insert over a PS. In the first step a tibial platform is restored with a trial component attached to an intramedullary stem extension. Stabilization of the flexion gap follows, where most of the important work is done: (a) correct rotation of femoral component, (b) size of femoral component to restore tension to collaterals when possible, and (c) evaluation of joint line height, usually with respect to the position of the inferior pole of the patella. If the arthroplasty is unstable in flexion even after the largest possible femoral component (extends from medial to lateral cortex) is paired with a thick PS insert, this demonstrates that collateral ligaments have failed and a CC component is required. This is the first indication for a CC in revision TKA.

The third step in the revision is simple: as the knee is extended, the selected tibial insert pushes the femoral component more proximally. When full extension is reached, the femoral trial component position is recorded and, in most systems, bone cuts can be made through the trial component to accommodate distal femoral augments that are typically between 5 and 10 mm thick. In this way we have matched the size of the extension gap to that of the flexion gap. The second indication for constraint, instability in extension secondary to ligament failure, will be obvious.

It has been my experience with this technique that a PS or CC insert can stabilize almost all cases. This includes structural allografts of the proximal tibia or distal femur as well as ligamentous reconstructions. Linked constrained devices (hinges) are an option for more severe degrees of the instability described here, but the hyperextension stop in most designs may increase loosening rates.

References

1. Vince KG, Abdeen A, Sugimori T. The unstable total knee arthroplasty: causes and cures. *J Arthroplasty.* 2006;21(4 Suppl 1):44-49.
2. Berger RA, et al. Malrotation causing patellofemoral complications after total knee arthroplasty. *Clin Orthop Relat Res.* 1998;(356):144-153.
3. Babis GC, Trousdale RT, Morrey BF. The effectiveness of isolated tibial insert exchange in revision total knee arthroplasty. *J Bone Joint Surg Am.* 2002;84-A(1):64-68.

HOW SHOULD I MANAGE THE PATIENT WITH CHRONIC EXTENSOR MECHANISM DEFICIENCY ASSOCIATED WITH A TOTAL KNEE ARTHROPLASTY?

R. Stephen J. Burnett, MD, FRCS(C)
Robert L. Barrack, MD

The patient that presents with a *chronically* deficient extensor mechanism (EM) is one of the most challenging clinical problems in association with TKA revision surgery. We define a deficiency as any extensor lag >30 degrees, in association with symptoms of instability as a result of a dysfunctional or disrupted EM. In our experience, this problem occurs infrequently, in the range of 0.1 to 2.5% of all primary and revision TKA procedures. Attempts at primary repair of the EM are unsuccessful in this chronic patient group, as the disruption typically has been present for >6 months.[1]

EM deficiency may be due to: patellar or quadriceps tendon avulsion/rupture; periprosthetic patella fracture; or fragmentation of the patella. Typically these disruptions are not recognized intraoperatively, but frequently some degree of drainage occurs intraoperatively. The disruption probably initiates intraoperatively and is completed in the course of therapy of ambulation and is often blamed on an event soon after surgery. We have identified several risk factors that may be associated with developing an EM deficiency following primary or revision TKA: obesity, females, patella infera and difficult exposure during TKA, recurrent extensile exposures, lateral retinacular releases, over resection of patellar bone during patella resurfacing, revision TKA surgery, and most recently, minimally invasive TKA surgery (MIS). Conversion/takedown of a prior knee fusion is an uncommon procedure for which we also use an extensor mechanism allograft (EMA).

While bracing is an option for patients that are not suitable to undergo further surgery, reconstruction with the use of an EMA in association with a TKA has been shown to have good clinical results at medium-term follow-up in several recently reported clinical series.[1-4]

Preoperatively, we always evaluate the patient for occult TKA infection with an ESR and CRP, and if these are elevated, an aspiration for synovial fluid nucleated cell count and culture is performed. In addition, if there has been radiographic patellar maltracking following the TKA, we obtain a CT scan of the knee to assess for tibial and femoral component malrotation, which requires component revision in addition to reconstruction of the EM. We ask our radiologist to use the technique and protocol described by Berger et al.[5]

Surgical options to reconstruct the chronically deficient EM include the use of allografts or an extended medial gastrocnemius rotational flap (EMGRF). An EMGRF is rarely used in our practice. This procedure can provide successful salvage of a failed extensor mechanism allograft or an alternative to allograft reconstruction in patients with poor soft tissue coverage, previous infection, or a compromised immune system. When we perform an EMGRF, we do so in conjunction with a plastic surgeon. This procedure has been described by Jaureguito et al,[6] and it is usually the *extended* version of the flap (that includes achilles tendon) that we use to reconstruct the patellar tendon.

More commonly, we use an EMA to reconstruct the deficient EM. There are two types of allograft tissue that you may require, depending on the anatomic location of the deficiency, and the remaining host EM tissues. We have used either a total extensor mechanism allograft of the knee (EMAK) (quadriceps tendon, patella, patellar tendon, and tibial tubercle) or, an achilles tendon-calcaneal bone block allograft (ATA) for reconstruction.[1] We use a simple algorithm to decide which of these two allografts we will require. The choice of graft depends on the location and status of the remaining patella, mobility of the quadriceps, and the status of the bone stock at the tibial tubercle. This algorithm attempts to maintain a viable portion of the host extensor mechanism, when appropriate, and we believe, most closely represents the problems that you will encounter. If the patella is retracted excessively and can not be mobilized to a position placing the patella within 2 to 3 cm of the joint line with the knee in extension (in the O.R., during the exposure), we use an EMAK. If the patella and patellar component are intact and can be mobilized within 2 to 3 cm of the joint line in extension, we retain the patella and use an ATA sewn to the quadriceps mechanism with the knee in full extension after the quadriceps is mobilized and placed under tension (Figure 46-1). If there is massive osteolysis, including the tibial tubercle, then an ATA is used, placing the calcaneal bone block distal to the area of the lytic lesion. If the patella is absent or insufficient, then we use an EMAK to help restore the lever arm of the patella. If we are performing a takedown of a knee fusion, we find that due to the chronic contracture of the anterior soft tissues and skin, an EMAK often "over stuffs" the anterior knee, making skin closure problematic, thus we recommend using an ATA when performing this procedure (Figure 46-2). Nonirradiated allograft (fresh-frozen) is preferred, although all of the allografts obtained typically have been irradiated at a low dose. We (and others)[1-4] never resurface the patella when using the EMAK.

Technical pearls of the procedure(s) are as important as the choice of allograft. These are best described in the attached references, with both schematic and intra-operative step-wise details for allografts and the EMGF.[1,7] Make sure you ask for a specimen that includes a minimum (or "…as much length as possible") of 4 cm of quadriceps tendon, and the entire tibia attached, or, a large calcaneal bone segment with the entire achilles tendon attached, and look at them in *advance* of your surgery. Revision of components, when necessary, should always be performed prior to the EMA reconstruction. Use a

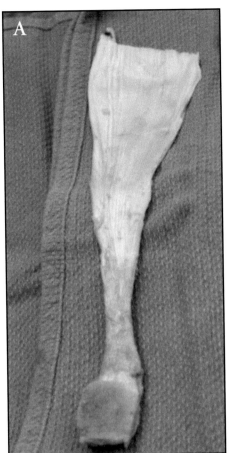
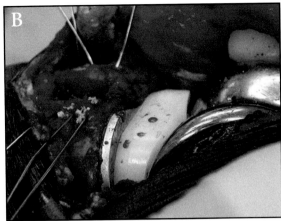
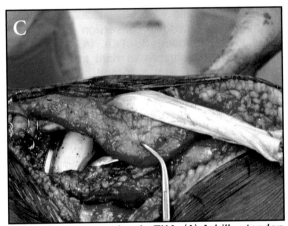

Figure 46-1. Technique of Achilles' tendon allograft reconstruction in TKA. (A) Achilles tendon fresh frozen allograft is harvested, with an attached calcaneal bone block. A generous bone block is later cut to size for the tibial insertion. (B) The host tibial trough is prepared to accept the allograft bone block. The trough is typically 1.5 cm width 2.5 cm length, and is just medial to the host tibial tubercle. We leave cancellous bone at the base of the cortical window to encourage healing and impact the allograft tubercle bone plug into the cancellous bed. To do this, the depth of the trough is usually only a few mm deep (<3 to 4 mm). The trough is created smaller than the allograft to allow for a press-fit of the slightly oversized allograft bone block. Three wires or cables are passed beneath the floor of the host tibial trough for allograft fixation. The allograft is tamped into place and the wires are tightened. (C) The allograft is passed through a slit in the lateral retinaculum (posterior and lateral) to host patellar tendon remnant, then pulled proximally anterior to the host patella. The allograft is tensioned and sewn into the host quadriceps mechanism with Ethibond suture.

slightly medialized host tibial bone block trough, and dove-tail your allograft tibial (or calcaneal) segment. Three #18 g wires, low-profile 2 mm cables, or small fragment 3.5 mm cortical screws (pelvic set) may be used for the fixation on the tibial side. We tension the allograft tightly in full extension when using an ATA. When using an ATA it is important to mobilize the quads but to not pull the patella to tightly distally to avoid patella baja. In full extension the patella should be pulled distally until it is about 1 cm proximal to the joint line. When using an EMAK we tension it tightly in 30 degrees of flexion to

DO YOU USE STATIC OR AN ARTICULATING SPACER FOR RESECTION ARTHROPLASTY PRIOR TO REIMPLANTATION?

Alexander Siegmeth, FRCS(Tr & Orth)
Donald Garbuz, MD, FRCSC

Despite advances in antibiotic prophylaxis and surgical technique, infection remains a persistent problem, with infection rates ranging between 0.5% and 2% for primary TKA. The two options for treatment of a late, chronic infection are single-stage and two-stage revision arthroplasty. Proponents of a single-stage approach quote an eradication rate of between 80% and 90%.[1] Advantages include a single procedure with reduced hospital stay and lesser costs (if eradication of the infection is successful). The two-stage protocol as popularized by Insall et al,[2] involves removal of the prosthetic components and associated cement along with debridement of any infected appearing tissue or bone followed by organism specific antibiotic treatment for several weeks. This is followed by a second stage reimplantation of new components once the infection has been eradicated.

A major disadvantage of the two-stage concept was that the interval between the two stages was associated with limited mobility, prolonged bed rest, and an oftentimes extended hospitalization. Immobility of the knee resulted in abundant scar formation within the joint and great difficulty with exposure at the time of re-implantation. Antibiotic loaded cement spacers were developed to address some of these limitations. In this technique, antibiotic loaded cement is placed into the knee joint to create a temporary knee fusion of sorts (Figure 47-1). These spacers deliver high local doses of antibiotics and hold the joint capsule and ligaments out to length thus facilitating exposure and reconstruction to some extent at the second stage; however, they do not allow the knee to bend. Problems encountered with these spacers, include instability with the potential for dislocation, damage to the patellar tendon and bone loss if relative motion occurs between the spacer and the host bone (Figure 47-2). In addition, exposure at the second stage is still difficult, often requiring an extensile exposure such as a quadriceps turndown or tibial tubercle osteotomy.

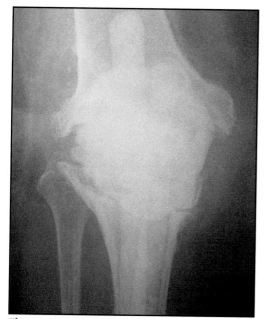

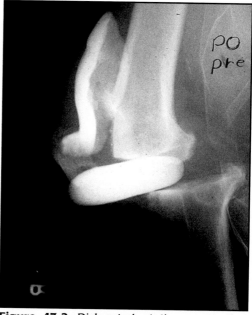

Figure 47-1. Static spacer.

Figure 47-2. Dislocated static spacer that damaged the patellar tendon.

Our unit developed the concept of articulating spacers with the prosthesis of antibiotic loaded acrylic cement (PROSTALAC). The PROSTALAC has evolved from a handmade facsimile of a knee prosthesis into a sophisticated system of molds with a posterior stabilized design. At the time of the first stage surgery, we remove the infected prosthesis including all cement; one of the most common causes of failure that we see is retained pieces of cement left behind at the time of the first stage resection arthroplasty. While we are meticulous when it comes to the debridement, we do take particular care to preserve as much bone at possible at the first stage so as to facilitate the second-stage reconstruction.

The bony surfaces of the tibia and femur are prepared for a standard revision knee arthroplasty. We approach the tibia first and after choosing a size that optimizes coverage of the upper end of the tibia, the thickness of the component fabricated is determined using spacer blocks (available sizes range from 12 to 34 mm). The component includes a polyethylene bearing surface and a cement post for the posterior stabilized design (Figure 47-3A). I add 3.6 g of Tobramycin and 1.5 g of Vancomycin to each package of cement that is used to make the spacer. Similar to the tibial component, most of the femoral component is made of antibiotic-loaded cement, however, the articular surface contains a low friction stainless steel bearing that articulates with the polyethylene of the tibial component (Figure 47-3B). A crossbar connects the two articulating halves and acts as the cam in the posterior stabilized design. Once the femoral component is sized, we can augment the distal femur and restore the joint line by increasing the thickness of the PROSTALAC femoral component; molds that produce three different thicknesses of the distal cement mantle are available for each size. Once the cement has hardened, the molds are removed. At this point, we mix another batch of antibiotic-loaded cement and loosely cement the

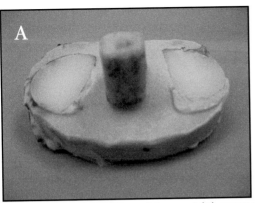
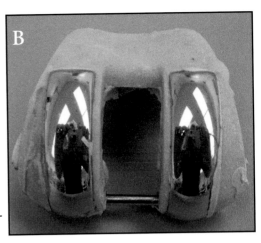

Figure 47-3. Tibial (A) and femoral (B) components of the PROSTALAC.

implants to the host bone at a later stage of polymerization to allow easier removal with less bone loss at the second stage; the tourniquet is deflated prior to final cementing to further impede interdigitation of the cement. We do not resurface the patella at the first stage.

Patients are allowed to toe touch weight bear until the second stage procedure and are allowed active and passive range of motion between stages. Our regimen includes 6 weeks of intravenous antibiotics at home prior to the second stage re-implantation.

The main advantage of the PROSTALAC knee system as my colleagues and I see it, is maintenance of the joint line, ligament tension, and the ability to maintain range of motion between stages. This facilitates the second stage reimplantation significantly as post-operative scarring is reduced to a degree that we almost never need to use an extensile approach to obtain adequate exposure. Most of the complications we had with the original design of the PROSTALAC were related to the extensor mechanism.[4]

Similar to static spacers the PROSTALAC system allows maximal local antibiotic concentration and delivery; however, the primary disadvantage of the PROSTALAC is cost as the prosthesis is discarded after the first stage and availability is limited. Although the particular device described by us is not FDA approved for use in the United States, similar systems of molds are available that create an articulating spacer without the polyethylene inserts in the tibia or the metal runners on the surface of the femoral component.

In summary, we recommend the use of an articulating antibiotic-loaded spacer such as the PROSTALAC over a traditional static cement spacer as it allows for improved mobility of the patient, range of motion exercises between stages, and ease of exposure at the second stage revision.

References

1. Goeksan SB, Freeman MAR. One-stage re-implantation for infected total knee arthroplasty. *J Bone Joint Surg Br.* 1992;74B:78-82.
2. Insall JN, Thompson FM, Brause BD. Two-stage re-implantation for the salvage of infected total knee arthroplasty. *J Bone Joint Surg Am.* 1983;65:1087-1098.
3. Duncan CP, Beauchamp C, Masri B. The antibiotic loaded joint replacement system; a novel approach to the management of the infected knee replacement. *J Bone Joint Surg Br.* 1992;74B(Suppl 111):296.

4. Haddad FS, Masri B, Campbell D, McGraw R, Beauchamp CP, Duncan CP. The PROSTALAC functional spacer in two-stage revision for infected knee replacements. *J Bone Joint Surg Br.* 2000;82B:807-811.
5. Fehring TK, Odum S, Calton TF, Mason JB. Articulating versus static spacers in revision total knee arthroplasty for sepsis: The Ranawat Award. *Clin Orthop.* 2000; (380):9-16.

WHAT ARE YOUR INDICATIONS FOR A KNEE FUSION?

Andrew A. Freiberg, MD

Arthrodesis of the knee is an excellent, definitive limb sparing procedure that I sometimes use in the treatment of a chronically infected unrevisable total knee arthroplasty that is associated with severe compromise of the soft tissue envelope and typically, the extensor mechanism.[1-3] In rare instances, knee arthrodesis is performed for treatment of post-traumatic arthritis (usually in the setting of severe bone loss combined with extensor mechanism loss), in combination with medical treatment for infectious arthritis (tuberculous or other fungal infections), or very rarely, in osteoarthritis in a young laborer. The stability of an arthrodesis significantly improves the success of local flap coverage, and there may be a lower risk of infection recurrence in the treatment of resistant organisms. Oftentimes, a knee fusion will avoid the need for amputation in the severely compromised limb.

The practical indications for knee arthrodesis include the medical factors mentioned earlier, and equally important, patient acceptance of a truly permanent stiff knee and the functional limitations that are associated with a knee that does not bend. I typically have patients wear a knee immobilizer or a cylinder cast prior to knee fusion to clearly demonstrate to them the functional limitations that they will experience once their knee is fused. Although conversion of a surgical fused knee to a total knee arthroplasty is sometimes possible, the complication rate (including recurrence of infection) is considered unacceptably high by most surgeons.

The technique I have utilized relies on the use of a modular titanium nail that is assembled from within the knee joint. This avoids the need for a hip incision, and allows for independently sized implants within the femur and tibia. Modular fusion nails give much greater rotational stability and yet still allow compression at the site of arthrodesis. Shorter locked nails have been complicated by periprosthetic fractures, an unacceptable rate of device dissociation and extreme difficulty with removal if required.

I typically perform a knee fusion in a staged fashion with the first stage including the removal of the infected knee implant (or infected native bone) along with a radical debridement of any infected-appearing tissues, placement of an antibiotic spacer, and 6 weeks of organism-specific intravenous antibiotics in an attempt to eradicate the infection. At the second stage, I further debride the knee and use total knee cutting guides to facilitate preparation of the bony surfaces. The femoral and tibial intramedullary canals are flexibly reamed—1.5 mm greater than the nominal nail diameter for the femoral implant and usually 1 mm greater for the tibia. The femoral implant is curved, and if the canal is not over-reamed, incarceration of the nail is very possible. The nail is assembled and locked from within the knee. The ideal position of a fused knee is 7 ± 5 degrees of valgus and 15 ± 5 degrees of flexion. A leg that is slightly short facilitates clearance of the ipsilateral foot during ambulation; if a large leg length discrepancy is unavoidable, a shoe-lift may be required postoperatively.

Postoperatively, a thin, long-leg fiberglass cast is applied and immediate weight bearing encouraged. I include the foot in the cast to prevent a high rotation force at the arthrodesis side. Fusion usually occurs by 6 weeks, although it may take several months in patients with severe bone loss where allograft bone was utilized.

Alternatives to the technique I have described include the use of an external fixator to avoid retained hardware. Monloateral fixators have been associated with a higher rate of failure and thus biplanar or circular external fixation is recommended. These devices, however, can be cumbersome for the patient and pin-tract infection is a persistent problem. Plate fixation (usually performed with two plates) is another alternative; however, the indwelling hardware can result in persistent infection and weight bearing must be limited. As previously mentioned an antegrade locked nail can also be used; however, this technique requires a second incision at the hip and can potential spread the infection up the femoral and down the tibial canals. Further, optimal fixation can be compromised as the diameters of the femoral and tibial canals are oftentimes disparate and thus the use of a nail with a uniform diameter can be problematic.

References

1. Arroyo JS, Garvin KL, Neff JR. Arthrodesis of the knee with a modular titanium intramedullary nail. *J Bone and Joint Surg Am.* 1997;79:26-34.
2. Macdonald JH, Agarwal S, Lorei MP, Johanson NA, Freiberg AA. Knee arthrodesis. *J Amer Acad Orthop Surgeons* 2006;14:154-163.
3. Waldman BJ, Mont MA, Payman KR, Freiberg AA, Windsor RE, Sculco TP, Hungerford DS. Infected total knee arthroplasty treated with arthrodesis using as modular nail. *Clin Orthop Relat Res.* 1999;367:230-237.

Case Example

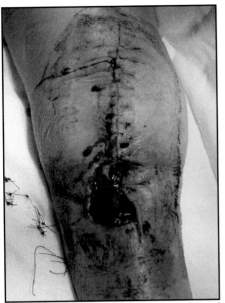

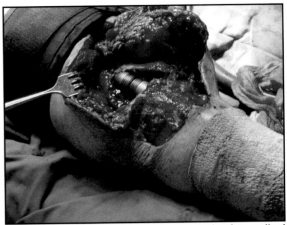

Figure 48-2. Intraoperative photograph after radical debridement and placement of modular, titanium fusion nail.

Figure 48-1. Patient with infected total knee, draining sinus, complete loss of extensor mechanism from two failed attempts at patellar tendon repair.

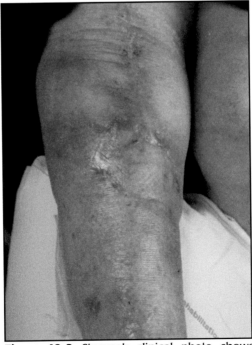

Figure 48-3. Six-week clinical photo shows healed gastrocnemius rotation flap and excellent cosmetic appearance of wound.

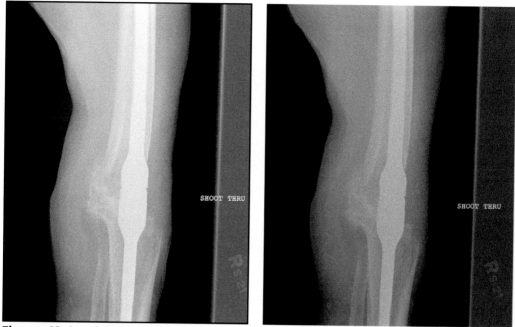

Figures 48-4 and 48-5. Radiographs at 6 weeks show healing of arthrodesis despite severe anterior bone loss.

HOW DO YOU MANAGE THE PATIENT WITH AN UNEXPECTEDLY POSITIVE CULTURE AT THE TIME OF A REVISION TOTAL KNEE ARTHROPLASTY?

Patrick M. Morgan, MD
John C. Clohisy, MD

Many surgeons performing a revision total knee arthroplasty for presumed aseptic loosening obtain intraoperative specimens for culture. If these specimens unexpectedly grow one or more culture can carry with it serious implications, interpretation of such a result must take a number of factors into account. The literature currently recognizes four distinct clinical scenarios that can produce a positive culture: (1) the unexpected positive intraoperative culture; (2) early postoperative infection; (3) late chronic infection, and (4) presumed acute hematogenous infection.[1] While there is a strong preference for operative management of the early, chronic, and acute hematogenous infections, the patient with an unexpected positive culture at the time of revision can oftentimes be managed with antibiotic therapy or even observation alone. In this clinical scenario, the patient's preoperative evaluation, appearance of the wound at the time of surgery, and tissue culture results are all factored into the treatment decision. Here, we describe our approach to the unexpected positive culture obtained during revision total knee arthroplasty.

Our pre-operative assessment for revision total knee patients includes a thorough history, physical examination, and radiographic evaluation. All patients are evaluated with laboratory studies including a complete blood cell count with differentials, an erythrocyte sedimentation rate, and a C-reactive protein. We routinely perform joint aspiration for cell count, differential, and culture as this test has been found to be particularly useful in identifying the colonized wound bed with a reported sensitivity, specificity, and accuracy of 75%, 96%, and 90%, respectively.[2] Suspicion for periprosthetic infection is increased in patients with a history of multiple surgeries and previous periprosthetic infection; patients with conditions such as rheumatoid arthritis, diabetes mellitus, chronic renal failure, human immunodeficiency virus, or a malignant tumor are considered to be potentially immunocompromised and are also evaluated with increased concern for occult sepsis. Technetium-99 m bone and isotope-labeled leukocyte scans are used in our practice on a very selective basis. We consider molecular techniques such as polymerase chain reaction investigational, and presently do not employ them for detecting occult infection.

The aforementioned pre-operative data is then used to stratify patients into three major groups. These are as follows: (1) *low risk* patients for whom our clinical suspicion for infection is low (a normal preoperative evaluation and a patient without risk factors for occult sepsis), (2) *moderate risk* patients have an equivocal preoperative work-up (patient with risk factors for occult sepsis or equivocal laboratory data with a negative knee aspirate culture), and (3) patients with a *documented infection*.

At the time of surgery, all patients undergoing revision total knee arthroplasty have at least five intra-articular biopsy specimens sent for culture from the most inflamed-appearing areas including samples from both the tibial and femoral canals.[3] Patients with a *low risk* of infection then undergo revision total knee arthroplasty. For patients with a *moderate risk* for infection specimens are sent intra-operatively for frozen section analysis before proceeding with prosthetic implantation. We use a threshold of five or more polymorphonuclear leukocytes per any high powered field, and patients at or above this threshold are treated with explanation and placement of an antibiotic-impregnated methacrylate spacer. Patients with a *documented infection* are most commonly treated with a two-stage knee reconstruction.

Intra-operative tissue culture can be plagued by false positive results. In one series, 30% of total hips undergoing revision for aseptic loosening had at least one positive intraoperative culture.[4] Of this group, however, only one patient later developed a clinically significant infection, indicating a high false-positive rate. Alternatively, a separate study showed isolation of an organism from three or more samples corresponded with confirmed septic loosening in 89% of cases.[5] Our bias trends toward clinical observation of one positive culture in patients with a *low risk* of active infection. Patients with one positive culture and *moderate risk* for infection are considered for antibiotic treatment and infectious disease consultation. When presented with two positive cultures of the same organism infectious disease consultation is obtained and antibiotic therapy strongly considered for both low and moderate risk patients (Table 49-1). The preoperative clinical concern for implant infection and the results of the intraoperative cultures are utilized to guide treatment decision making. "Treatment" refers to intravenous antibiotic therapy and infectious disease consultation. In cases of three or more positive intraoperative cultures the patient is assumed to have been reimplanted into a colonized wound bed and is treated accordingly. When indicated, treatment for both low and moderate risk patients involves the administration of appropriate intravenous antibiotic for 6 weeks and consultation with an infectious disease specialist. Using this protocol, infection has been reported to be eradicated in up to 90% of cases.[1] In the uncommon case of multiple positive cultures (3 or more), chronic antibiotic suppression may also be considered depending on the overall clinical situation.

Table 49-1
Treatment in the Face of Unexpected Positive Intraoperative Culture

Risk Stratification	*All Cultures Negative*	*One Positive Culture*	*Two or More Positive Cultures*
Low risk	No treatment	Observation	Treatment
Moderate risk	No treatment	• Consider antibiotic therapy • Infectious disease consultation	Treatment

References

1. Tsukayama DT, Estrada R, Gustilo RB. Infection after total hip arthroplasty. A study of the treatment of one hundred and six infections. *J Bone Joint Surg Am.* 1996;78:512-523.
2. Barrack RL, Jennings RW, Wolfe MW, Bertot AJ. The value of preoperative aspiration before total knee revision. *Clin Orthop.* 1997;345:8-16.
3. Kamme C, Lindberg L. Aerobic and anaerobic bacteria in deep infections after total hip arthroplasty: differential diagnosis between infectious and non-infectious loosening. *Clin Orthop.* 1981;154:201-207.
4. Padget DE, Sliverman A, Sachjowicz F, Simpson RB, Rosenberg AG, Galante JO. Efficacy of intraoperative cultures obtained during revision total hip arthroplasty. *J Arthroplasty.* 1995;10:420-426.
5. Pandey R, Berendt AR, Athanasou NA. Histological and microbiological findings in non-infected revision arthroplasty tissues. The OSIRIS Collaborative Study Group. Oxford Skeletal Infection Research and Intervention Service. *Ach Orthop Trauma Surg.* 2000;120:570-574.

INDEX

Achilles tendon, use of for allograft for extensor mechanism disruptions, 139–140

Achilles tendon-calcaneal bone block allograft. *See* ATA

activity level, effect of on surgical options, 9

allograft prosthetic composite, use of following supracondylar femur fractures, 136

allografts, structural, use of in revisions with massive bone loss, 174–175

angiogram, vascular injury after TKA and performance of, 119

ankle-brachial index, 16
use of to determine ischemia, 119

anterior knee pain, patella resurfacing and, 27–28

anterior referencing guides, femoral component sizing and, 75

anterior trochlear, gender differences in, 54

anterior-posterior axis, femoral component rotation and, 59–60

anteromedial release, during TKA in patients with varus deformity, 84

anti-notch guide, femoral component sizing and, 74

antibiotic cement. *See also* PROSTALAC
indications for use of, 105–106
precautions, 107
preparation of, 106–107
use of in two-stage revision arthroplasty, 199

arterial complications, risk factors for, 120

arthritis
nonoperative alternatives for, 3
operative decisions based on radiographic evidence of, 4

arthrodesis, indications for, 203–204

articulating spacers, 200–201
prefabricated, use of for periprosthetic joint infection, 107

aspirin, use of for DVT prophylaxis, 117

ATA, use of to repair chronic extensor mechanism deficiency, 194–195

augments, use of for bone loss, 173–174

autologous blood donation, effects on hemoglobin of, 19–21

avascular necrosis
following patellar resection, 99
following patellar resurfacing, 28

balanced gaps, 31–32

bilateral TKA
blood management and, 20–21
one-stage vs. staged, 23–24

blood management, bilateral TKAs and, 20–21

bone grafts, use of for bone loss, 173

bone loss
methods of reconstruction for, 173
patellar, revision TKA and, 181–183

bupivacaine, intraoperative capsule injection of for perioperative pain management, 109–110